THE

SMALL

PATIENT

PRACTICE

2nd Edition

The Small Patient Practice

2nd Edition

A Beginner's Guide to Starting

A Pediatric PT, OT or SLP

Solo Practice

Including Medical Documentation,

Billing and Coding

Jeanine Gregoire Colburn

PT, DPT MS, PCS

Three Leaf Press

Three Leaf Press
97 Woodbridge Drive
Colorado Springs, CO 80906

For information regarding special discounts for bulk purchase, please
contact Three Leaf Press at 3leafpress@gmail.com

Manufactured in the United States of America

ISBN 978-0-9835033-2-3

A note to the Reader
This publication contains the opinions and ideas of its author. It is intended to provide helpful and
informative material on the subjects addressed in the publication. Although the author and publisher
have made every effort to ensure the accuracy and completeness of information contained in this
book, we assume no responsibility for errors, inaccuracies, omissions, or any inconsistency herein.
This publication is not intended for use as a source of legal or accounting advice. The publisher wants
to stress that the information contained herein may be subject to varying state and/or local laws or
regulations. All users are advised to retain competent counsel to determine what state and/or local
laws or regulations may apply to user's particular business.
The Purchaser or Reader of this publication assumes responsibility for the use of these materials and
information. Adherence to all applicable laws and regulations, federal, state, and local, governing
professional licensing, business practices, and all other aspects of doing business in the United States
is the sole responsibility of the Purchaser or Reader.
Any perceived slights of people or organizations are unintentional.

First printing 2017

To all of the wonderful

Pediatric

Physical therapists,

Occupational therapists,

and

Speech-Language Pathologists

With whom I have

Shared my career

Table of Contents

INTRODUCTION 1

   The Small Patient Practice 1

Chapter 1: 3

A Medical Billing and Documentation Guide for Pediatric Rehabilitation Therapists 3

   Just tell me what to do so I can get paid! 3

   Getting Started 5

   Next Steps 8

Chapter 2: 11

Understanding Your Patient's Healthcare Plan 11

   Contact Your Patient's Insurance Company 12

   Pros and Cons of Network Service Provision 14

   Invitations to Join a Network 16

Chapter 3: 17

Required and Recommended Elements of a Patient Record File 17

   Required Documents to Keep on File 19

   Recommended Medical Record Documentation 22

Chapter 4: 25

Documentation 25

   The Evaluation 26

   The Re-evaluation 33

   Progress Report 33

   Treatment Note 34

   Discharge Note 37

Chapter 5: 41

Billing for Outpatient Pediatric Rehabilitation Services 41

   The Claim Form 41

Chapter 6: 55

Coding for Diagnoses and Services 55

   ICD 10 Codes 55

   CPT Codes 59

   Coding Modifiers and Special Circumstances 65

Chapter 7...71

Those Dang PT and OT Evaluation Codes...71

    Required Elements of the Physical Therapy Evaluation.......................72

    Required Elements of the Occupational Therapy Evaluation...............76

Chapter 8:..81

Reading the Explanation of Benefits (EOB)..81

    An EOB with No Payment..81

    More Information Needed..82

    Amount Allowed...82

    Amount Allowed vs. Amount Paid...82

    Amount Paid vs Amount Billed...83

    Coinsurance vs Copayment...83

    One Common Mistake...83

Chapter 9:..87

Billing the Patient..87

    Balance Billing..87

    Consistent Billing...88

    Cash Based Practice..88

    How to Bill the Patient for Copayments and Deductibles...................88

    Reducing Patient Cost..89

    Patient Refusal to Pay..89

Chapter 10:..91

Wording Your Medical Records...91

    Developmental Delay...92

    Sensory Integration..93

    Progressive Disorders..93

Chapter 11:..97

Troubleshooting...97

    Patient Needs Adaptive Equipment..97

    Patient's Healthcare Policy has a Restricted Number of Visits per Year for Service..........98

    Health Insurance Payer Denies Payment..98

    Reimbursement is Delayed...100

    The Healthcare Payer Wants Reimbursement...................................100

Policy Denies Payment Because Child Getting Services in School 101

Payer Policy Does Not Cover Reported Service 102

Payer Reimbursement is Insufficient 102

CHAPTER 12: 105

Your Office, Your Practice and HIPAA 105

Health Information Privacy 106

FAX 108

Phone 109

Scheduling 109

Reliability 110

No Shows 110

Parent Not Present for Appointment 110

Coordinating Services With Early Intervention Agencies 111

Paying Yourself 112

ACKNOWLEDGMENTS 115

Appendices and Password 117

Appendix A 119

Appendix B 121

Appendix C 123

Appendix D 125

Appendix E 127

Appendix F 129

Appendix G 131

Appendix H 133

Appendix I 135

Appendix J 137

Appendix K 139

Appendix L 141

Appendix M 143

Appendix N 145

Appendix O 147

GLOSSARY AND DEFINITIONS 149

INDEX 155

INTRODUCTION

The Small Patient Practice

The purpose of this book is to take the mystery out of medical insurance billing for Pediatric Physical Therapists, Occupational Therapists and Speech Language Pathologists. It is targeted toward solo practitioners who want to see private patients. However, any provider will find useful information for billing and documentation, as well as an understanding of how to meet industry standards and requirements in a cost effective way.

Changes in coding have occurred since the first edition of this book was published in 2011. There are also updated requirements for patient health information security. As a result, a second edition of this book was warranted. The basic information is the same as in the first edition. The rules for billing and coding have not changed. But technology is changing and so the requirements for security have been updated. Furthermore, since we have moved to the ICD 10 coding system, payers as well as providers are trying to decide how best to use and understand the codes. There have also been some changes in required procedural codes (CPT codes) that require some additional attention. With the expansion of telehealth service provision, additional codes and modifiers have been added.

I must have always known that I would be writing a second edition of this book. Over the years I have been contacted by various readers requesting additional clarification or explaining special circumstances that required my assistance. I saved those email requests and made sure to include the topics addressed in this new edition. The website **www.smallpatientpractice.com** provides an opportunity for readers to contact me. Additionally, as requested, I have added a page to that website that includes downloadable forms and charts that are in the appendices of this book. The user name and password for accessing downloads are in the appendices.

I have billed for services provided as a solo practitioner intermittently throughout my career. I have been a practicing physical therapist since 1975, but the first time I had to do my own billing was in 1991. When you move to a place that doesn't have the work opportunities you would prefer, sometimes you just have to create your own opportunities. I know that many therapists have been pressured into doing their own billing simply because state regulations have changed requiring health insurance to be accessed prior to using state early intervention funds. I actually billed health insurance for early intervention related physical therapy in 1991 simply because at that time my community EI program in New Mexico had no money to pay for therapists. They were looking for volunteers. I don't mind volunteering, but I would rather be paid for my professional work, if possible. In 1993, I moved to Virginia and was able to bill insurance for EI physical therapy there as well. Now I live in Colorado. At this writing I work part-time for an early intervention agency that bills health insurance and I see patients privately and do my own insurance billing.

I have been an active member of the American Physical Therapy Association throughout my career. I have found it to be a wonderful professional resource. The Academy of Pediatric Physical Therapy provides great continuing education opportunities and I just love interacting with fellow pediatric therapists. As of this writing, I currently serve on the Committee for Payment, Policy and Advocacy. This has given me the opportunity to learn therapist concerns and to get a sense of what is happening throughout the country in the world of billing and reimbursement. While researching information needed for this book, I discovered that the AOTA and ASHA websites are also wonderful resources.

As scary as it might seem, once you learn the rules and meet your local requirements for self-employment, you really don't have to focus on billing and administration. You really can focus on being the therapist you want to be. You will take care of your practice and provide the quality of care that your patients deserve.

This guide will help you understand requirements for medical billing and documentation. Furthermore, it will give you the tools to help you stay up to date with policy changes as they arise. I am presenting this material from a solo practitioner pediatric therapist perspective, but it should help any pediatric PT, OT or SLP learn the essentials of medical documentation, billing and coding. It is the culmination of what I have learned over the years and it will hopefully simplify the process for you.

Chapter 1:

A Medical Billing and Documentation Guide for Pediatric Rehabilitation Therapists

Just tell me what to do so I can get paid!

This is the first thing therapists want to know---so we will start with this and get to the details and explanations later in the book. Since it is my intent to take the mystery out of medical billing and documentation, I will give you everything up front. The detailed explanations and justifications will be in later chapters.

Keep in mind that the guidance in this book is not just a 'good idea', in most cases industry rules and regulations require compliance. The Health Insurance Portability & Accountability Act (HIPAA) requires providers and payers to comply with coding guidelines of the American Medical Association CPT (Current Procedural Terminology) Procedure codes and the International Classification of Disease, 10th Revision Clinical Modification diagnosis codes (ICD 10 codes). Payment policies are usually based on CPT descriptors. Furthermore, these code sets are to be maintained and are valid within the dates specified by their respective responsible organizations.[1] That means, if the ICD 10 coding or the CPT code

---

[1] Health Insurance Portability and Accountability Act of 1996 (HIPAA); 45 United States Code § 1320d et seq.; Part C Administrative Simplification.

guidelines are officially changed, then you are obliged to follow the new rules as written within the dates of implementation.

Documentation rules are defined in the Policy Manuals available on the Centers for Medicare and Medicaid website. [2] Even if you don't see Medicare or Medicaid patients, most public and private insurance payers default to the CMS rules as they are readily available and transparent.

Many pediatric therapists have worked in schools and Early Intervention programs which prefer documentation in a 'non-medical' format. Now, after years of communicating in a family friendly and non-problem oriented manner, pediatric therapists are asked to put their medical hats back on in order to access medical funding for their services. This isn't difficult. You know your profession. It is just a different means of communicating.

Does Health Care Reform affect this information?

Health Care Reform is more 'policy' oriented. This book is geared toward the details of billing and documentation.   The information provided in this book has been the industry standard for a number of years. The rules for documentation and billing have changed very little for our profession. I have been a physical therapist for more than 40 years and only this year has coding and rules for the physical therapy evaluation changed. In my opinion, electronic billing and HIPAA standards have had the greatest effect on reimbursement. In the past, some private payers and even state Medicaid programs did not use publicly available coding guidelines and sometimes even created their own codes or changed the reimbursement rules around particular codes. This proved to be very confusing to providers. Electronic billing has caused payers to realign their reimbursement policies to comply with HIPAA guidelines. Now payers may use available automated programs to process electronic payments and recognize irregularities in billing. This prevents providers from billing incorrectly and likely saves the payers a lot of money. The value of this is that as providers, we only need to learn one set of billing and reimbursement rules. The drawback is that you may not be able to be as flexible in your coding as you may prefer.

---

45 Code of Federal Regulations, Parts 160, 162, and 164 ("Privacy Rule")

[2] http://www.cms.hhs.gov/

It is important to realize that various healthcare reimbursement organizations will occasionally change their policies around reimbursement or coverage. This has been going on for years and will continue. Although this may affect a particular aspect of the service you provide, it rarely affects the administrative side of your practice.

Getting Started

Be a qualified Physical Therapist, Occupational Therapist or Speech-Language Pathologist.

You have already paid for the most costly portion of your practice if you are a qualified rehabilitation therapist.

Physical Therapist must be licensed in the state in which she/he is practicing unless licensure does not apply, graduated from an approved or accredited Physical Therapy education program and passed a national examination approved by the state in which PT services are provided.

Occupational Therapist is licensed or otherwise regulated as an OT in the state in which practicing. If licensure or other regulation does not apply, the OT has graduated from an OT education program accredited by ACOTE or the AMA and AOTA and is eligible to take, or has successfully completed the NBCOT examination for Occupational Therapists.

Speech-Language Pathologist is licensed or if licensure or other regulation does not apply, must have the education and experience requirements for a Certificate of Clinical Competence in speech-language pathology granted by the American Speech-Language Hearing Association or meet the educational requirements for certification and is in the process of accumulating the supervised experience required for certification. Some states have or are working toward licensure requirements.[3]

Basically, if you are a licensed medical provider in your state, then you are qualified to provide medical services. If your state does not have licensure for your profession, then you should abide by the above guidelines and your state Medicaid policies for provider qualifications. Keep in mind that Public School policies regarding the qualification of service providers do not always meet the standards for medical service provision. However, you must always meet your professional guidelines and licensure rules for service provision, regardless of setting.

Get Liability Insurance.

Your professional association is the place to look for liability insurance. If you are planning to work less than 20 hours a week, you may qualify for a discount. I think the price is reasonable, especially with the discounted rate for part time work. Don't begin seeing patients as a solo practitioner until you have this in place. If you already have liability insurance, but purchased it as an employed therapist, you should contact your plan and make certain you have coverage as a solo practitioner.

Get an NPI number.

This is free. Go to https://nppes.cms.hhs.gov/NPPES for a National Provider Identifier. This will be your unique health care provider identifier for electronic billing. If your office is in your home, you will give your home address as your practice or business location, even if you plan to see patients in their homes. Your practice location is the location of your office. You should have your new number within a couple of days of your application. If you have been working for another practice, it is possible that you already have an NPI number assigned to your name. You can check to see if you already have a number at this same website. You use this same number whether it was being used when you worked in another setting or when

---

[3] http://www.cms.hhs.gov/manuals/Downloads/bp102c15.pdf If you would like more details on the qualifications for service providers, go to this document and scroll down to sections 230.1, 230.2 and 230.3.

you work on your own. The only time you would request a different NPI number would be if you decided to expand to a group practice in the future.

Check on state and local regulations regarding private practices.

If you are planning to see patients in their homes, you will need to make sure you don't need any special licenses or permissions, or if you do, you must do what is necessary to comply. Most states do not require additional licenses unless you have a group practice or employees, then you may have to meet special requirements. For instance, in Colorado, we can see patients in their homes as solo practitioners without any additional license other than our professional license. However, if we provide service as a group of two or more, the Department of Health and Environments requires that we obtain an additional 'Home Care' license. Your state professional association may be able to advise you on any special requirements in your state. If you are planning to provide services in your home office, you should be certain there are no special ordinances or neighborhood restrictions, and if there are, make certain you are able to comply with those. Check your city and county ordinances, as well as neighborhood covenants. There are huge variations on these issues from state to state and even county to county. In most cases, these permissions or licenses are not very costly. You just need to make sure you have notified the local authorities, if required, that you have a business in your home.

Incorporate or not?

Whether to incorporate or not is up to you. Sometimes a particular payer may require incorporation. Most payers simply require you to have the proper licenses and permissions. If incorporation is not required, your decision will be determined by your personal and current financial status and whether you need additional protections. There are costs involved with incorporating and the tax structure of your income will change slightly. I suggest you speak to your tax accountant and weigh the pros and cons.

Depending upon the state you live in, you may have a choice in the type of corporation. There are Professional Corporations (PC) and Limited Liability Corporations (LLC) and others. Instead of incorporating you can also practice under a Business License with the name of your choosing. Your state government website will have information on your options with definitions and rules.

So you are ready!

If you are a qualified PT, OT or SLP, have liability insurance, an NPI number and have the necessary local permissions, **you are ready to bill health care insurance for your services.**

Next Steps

There is no need to try to become a network provider for every known insurance company. That would be impossible and in most cases, not necessary. If I am contacted by a patient with a new insurance, I will contact the insurance company and find out about that patient's particular plan.

1. Contact the patient's healthcare insurance and ask about the plan.
This will help you determine if you can begin seeing the patient immediately and bill for your services, or if you will need to pursue a network contract or some other form of permission. In Chapter 2, I will go into more detail regarding gathering the insurance information you will need toward determining next steps. I will also discuss things you may want to consider before deciding whether to be a network provider and what this means. If you are ready to begin seeing the patient, you need to set up a patient file.

2. Set up a patient record file.
This will help you stay organized and keep all relevant patient information and documents in one place. In Chapter 3, 'Required and Recommended Elements of a Patient Record File and Meeting HIPAA Regulations', I will give you more detail regarding the required elements of a patient record. Keep in mind that if you have a home office you are still required to take the necessary steps to protect patient privacy. You should have a locking file cabinet and your computer should have protections which will prevent unauthorized access to private information. Patient privacy protections will be discussed further in Chapter 3 as well as in Chapter 12.

3. Evaluate the patient and determine your plan of care

Your evaluation and plan of care are the keys to success. This is not a School Based or Early Intervention oriented 'evaluation' where you are simply determining if the child meets state criteria to qualify for publicly funded services. Those evaluations are typically standardized developmental evaluations with numeric cutoffs, or broad determinations of disabilities and impairments. A medically oriented outpatient therapy evaluation must determine if there is an underlying pathology which is treatable within a predictable period of time. For instance, a physical therapist does not treat Down Syndrome, but does treat muscle weakness or difficulty walking, regardless of whether the child has Down Syndrome. Chapter 4, 'Documentation' will go into detail regarding defensible documentation.

4. Determine your method of billing for this patient's services.

There are several options here. Don't let anyone tell you that you should purchase an expensive electronic documentation and billing program. These programs are set up for high volume practices with multiple coding options. They are cool and convenient, but a solo pediatric rehabilitation therapist has very limited coding options and cannot see the volume of patients in a given week which would justify the need for such a program. Many insurance companies have their own online billing program. Sometimes they are set up only for network providers, but sometimes you simply need to sign up for a login and password. Paper bills are always an option and sometimes required. There are also publicly accessible electronic billing programs. Many are cost-free. Details will be provided in Chapter 5, 'Billing for Outpatient Pediatric Rehabilitation Services'.

5. Determine which ICD 10 codes and CPT codes support your evaluation of the patient's needs and your plan of care.

Often ICD 10 and CPT codes are the thing that most worry therapists. How do you find these codes? How do you decide what to use? Chapter 6 'Coding for Diagnoses and Services' will discuss this in detail.

6. Complete the claim form and submit

Note that anything you put on the form, whether on paper or electronically, is your promise that the information you provided is true and accurate. Mistakes happen all the time, so you can always correct your claim. Keep in mind that mistakes are time intensive to correct and it is better to get it right the first time. See Chapter 5, 'Billing for Outpatient Pediatric Rehabilitation Services'. Be certain your patient care documentation supports your billing. See Chapter 4 'Documentation'. Keep in mind that insurance companies just want to know who the patient is, who you are and what services you are billing. The guidelines help us all to communicate in a uniform manner.

When You Get Paid or Receive a Statement from the Payer

The EOB or 'Explanation of Benefits' provides very important information and you can learn a lot from the information provided. Some EOBs are easier to read and more informative than others. The EOB will tell you if you need to bill the patient for any additional amount. It will also tell you if the insurance company needs additional information. See Chapter 8, Reading the Explanation of Benefits (EOB).

You Are Required to Bill the Patient/Family for Copayments and Deductibles

If the copayment is a flat rate per visit, you can collect the payment at the time of each visit. If the insurance plan requires a 'coinsurance' which is usually a percentage of the amount allowed or billed, you will need to bill the patient once you receive the EOB and verify the amount. There are variations depending upon whether you are an in-network or non-network provider. You will get this information in Chapter 9, 'Billing the Patient'.

That's it!

You are now a solo practitioner with the capability to bill various payers as you desire.

Read on for detailed information on billing, coding, documentation, resources and examples.

Chapter 2:

Understanding Your Patient's Healthcare Plan

There are hundreds of healthcare insurance companies in the United States. Within each company several plans are available to the patient. A healthcare insurance will have company policies that apply to all plans and then each plan will have its own policies. The policies within each plan will affect cost, provider access and rules around services.

Additionally, there are privately funded plans which are completely covered by an employer for its employees. These privately funded plans are tailored to the desires of the company, but may be administered by a public company, such as Cigna. You will not know the elements of a patient's plan specific to your service until you call and ask.

Medicaid is a state run healthcare plan with federal and state funding. Although the federal government provides guidelines for implementation of Medicaid, each state has considerable leeway in the implementation of the program. The intent of Medicaid is to provide healthcare access for people with low income. Most state Medicaid plans additionally provide funding for children with disabilities in some fashion. Your state Medicaid program may not be called 'Medicaid'. Your state professional organization can point you in the right direction. It is possible that your state Medicaid program will not cover your service. Every state is different.

As a solo practitioner pediatric rehabilitation provider you do not need to know everything about every plan. All you really need to know is whether your potential patient's plan covers outpatient Physical Therapy, or Occupational Therapy, or Speech Language-Pathology, whether there are specific parameters and whether you will be able to bill that insurance for your service.

Contact Your Patient's Insurance Company

Before contacting a potential patient's health care plan, you will need the following information: the patient's name, date of birth (DOB), Medical ID number and if applicable, the sponsor's name, DOB and Medical ID number. The 'sponsor' is the primary 'insured' in the plan, usually a parent, in the case of children. But sometimes there is no sponsor and the child is the sole insured, as would be the case in a Medicaid plan. You can find this information on the patient's medical insurance card. At times, however, your initial patient contact will be by phone and you will need to gather the information manually. The patient or patient's family can give you the insurance plan phone number.

In Appendix A, you will find a form labeled *Intake Insurance Information*. This is the form I use when I am getting insurance information from the patient. If you can get the information online or by fax, just print it and include it in the patient record.

When calling the insurance company, be sure to specify that you are requesting information regarding OUTPATIENT PHYSICAL THERAPY or OUTPATIENT OCCUPATIONAL THERAPY or OUTPATIENT SPEECH THERAPY. If you are planning to see the patient in the home, do not say this when you call about benefits or you may not get the information you need. The benefits person who answers the phone could get confused and think you are requesting home healthcare services. See below.

A special note about outpatient therapy provided in the patient's home. First, you need to understand that outpatient therapy services may be furnished in the therapist's office or in the patient's home.[4] Most medical insurance companies have policies which require them to align their policies with those of Medicare. So if you ever are challenged regarding your location of service, first look up the Medicare

---

[4] Medicare Benefit Policy manual, Pub 100-02, chapter 15, 230.4

rule listed on the footnote at the bottom of the page to verify the policy is still true, then share it with the payer and, at least in my experience, that will take care of the question. Better yet, sometimes the insurance company will state the policy as one of its own and you can refer the person challenging the service to his or her own company policy. Generally, I try not to mention my location of service to the person who answers the phone when I am calling about patient benefits. If the person you speak to happens to ask directly for location of service, that person just wants to know your office address. The location of service is properly documented during billing. Home Healthcare Agencies use PT, OT and Speech Therapy treatment codes that are specifically designated for home healthcare services. The treatment codes you will use are outpatient therapy codes, so there is usually no confusion once you actually bill for your services.

Here is what you need to ask the insurance company:

Does the plan allow your outpatient service?

What are the rules and restrictions around your service?

Does the payer allow an unlimited number of visits per year based on need? Or, are there restrictions in number of visits per profession or combination of professions?)

Does the plan allow non-network service provision? (If you do not have a contract with that company, then you are a non-network service provider.)

What are the copayments and deductibles in network and out of network for your service?

What is the insurance coverage year start date? (This is important---most start on January 1, but some start on October 1 and others start on July 1. The start date of the insurance year means the deductible amount starts all over again.)

I created an information form to help me to remember all pertinent questions when calling the insurance company. See Appendix B and look at the form labeled *Patient Insurance Plan Data*. Feel free to use it yourself or use it as a model to create one of your own.

Once you have gathered the needed information, you can determine if you will first need a network contract in place prior to providing and billing for services, whether you need a prior authorization from the insurance company in order to be reimbursed for your services, or if you can provide and bill for services for this patient right away.

Pros and Cons of Network Service Provision

It is not always in your patient's best interest to become a network service provider. Plans and rules can vary greatly for network versus non-network services. You should consider many factors when deciding whether to be a network provider.

If a healthcare insurance company provides coverage for a major segment of your community population, you may want to pursue a network contract, especially if a network contract is required for service provision.

There is a huge variation in the rules and policies around network contracts. Some contracts will be good for you and the patient. Some will be good for you but not the patient. Some will be good for the patient but not for you.

The issue of getting referrals is not usually a pediatric therapist concern as most communities have a shortage in pediatric therapists. It is important to consider whether the patient's insurance plan allows access to your services or those of another pediatric therapist in your community. Hopefully the patient can see at least one of you.

Here are some situations you may run into:

1. Sometimes it may be unreasonable or impossible for a pediatric therapist to become a network provider for an insurance plan, but the plan will provide a non-network authorization for your services to your patient, since there are no pediatric therapists in the network. (When I say it may be unreasonable to become a network provider, it is usually because the network policies and reimbursement rules are clearly set up for the adult orthopedic population and it would be too costly or cumbersome for a pediatric therapist to be a network provider).

2. Some insurance plans, especially self-funded plans, may not have network plans. So there is no requirement to be a network provider. These plans may or may not require prior authorization for your services. Once you bill for

your services, be prepared to submit a copy of a W-9 (tax form) on request, or a copy of the doctor referral, evaluation or treatment notes if requested.

3. Some benefit plans, especially government supported plans such as CHP[5], Medicaid and Tricare will only allow service provision from network providers. In these cases, you must pursue a network contract if you want to provide services to this patient population, or expect a substantial reduction in payment.

4. With many insurance plans, the patient will save money if you are a network provider. For instance, the network annual deductible may be $500, but the non-network annual deductible may be $1500. This isn't the only thing you should consider. Read on.

5. Sometimes the visit cost share for the patient is better if you are a non-network provider. For example, the patient may have a flat copayment of $35 per visit for network provider therapy visits and a 20% coinsurance for non-network services. To keep it simple, let's say that each visit charge is $100. If the payer allows $100 for network and non-network services, the patient share of costs would $35 if you are a network provider and $20 if you are a non-network provider. It would clearly be better for the patient if you were a non-network provider. Now, it is not usually this simple, but as you can see, you need to look at everything with an eye toward what you will be billing and how many visits you will provide. In addition to per visit cost, you should consider total out of pocket cost for the year when comparing the two. But remember that total out of pocket cost includes other healthcare services as well.

6. Some insurance plans are trying some creative methods of cutting costs with network contracts. For instance, the insurer may want to pay a flat rate per visit. However, the reimbursement rate may not be sufficient to cover the cost of service. In this case you may determine that you cannot afford to provide services as a network provider for that company, but you may still be able to

---

[5] CHP stands for Child Health Plan, some states call it CHIP (Child Health Insurance Program). It may go by other names as well. This is healthcare for children whose family income is too high to qualify for Medicaid, but who cannot access affordable healthcare.

provide services as a non-network provider with reimbursement at expected levels.

The point of introducing the above scenarios is to caution you to call the patient's insurance plan **before** providing service. Make certain you understand all of the rules and exceptions. If a prior authorization is required, make certain you know what the insurance company needs from you for the authorization. Usually everything can be faxed to the appropriate person.

In any case, do not plan on being a network provider for everyone. As a solo provider, it would just be too cumbersome. Consider the population in your community, who are the major payers and then on a case by case basis decide whether you want to pursue an additional network contract.

Invitations to Join a Network

On occasion you may be contacted by a 'network' administrator asking you to join their network. The company may actually be a middleman that may or may not be useful to you. Read the contract carefully. The advantage of some of these companies is that they may be connected to several healthcare payers, even payers you don't have a direct network agreement with, but the middleman will process your bill as a network provider. So being a network provider with one of these companies may connect you with other payers. The company may also process your bills more quickly than the primary payers, but your reimbursement will be a little less. The important thing is to just watch all of your payers. Look at reimbursement, look at the amount of time and energy required to get reimbursement, etc. You can always end network agreements if you decide that a payer requires too much energy on your part or that reimbursement is not sufficient. Also, you may find that reimbursement is better for you and the patient's family if you are not in network. Just pay attention and as you go along you can refine your program as needed.

Chapter 3:

Required and Recommended Elements of a Patient Record File

A patient record is necessary for your protection as a medical provider. It will include required documents and provide proof of service provision. The patient is entitled to have complete copies of his/her medical record and the patient may request that you share your evaluations and treatment notes with other medical providers. Your records may be subpoenaed to provide information in a court case.

The type of folder or document holder you use is up to you. It is difficult to get away from paper, but many of my colleagues have switched to completely electronic documentation. I have a combination of both but am progressively moving toward keeping everything electronically on my desktop. If you work from your home, archiving is much simpler electronically. Manila folders will work, but it is a little tricky to stay organized this way. I have used pocket folders and I have used the traditional medical document holder with the two-hole punch at the top with dividers. When the patient is discharged, I previously transferred the documents to a manila folder for archiving. On my desktop I archive patient files by year of discharge. There are likely better organized methods of doing this.

Electronic healthcare files are gaining popularity. Most of the currently available electronic health file programs are stored online making them easily available. I don't recommend investing a large amount of money in a system, especially if you only see a couple of patients. Most available systems are still not adapted to the needs of a small practice pediatric rehabilitation provider at this time. Hopefully in the future the cost will decrease. Of course you can always create your own desktop file system for your medical records. Just be certain you have a backup system in place.

HIPAA has updated guidelines for the protection of electronically stored patient information. Keep in mind that one of the most common vulnerabilities of exposure to protected health information (PHI) is through the loss or theft of an unprotected laptop or cell phone. HIPAA rules dictate that any device with PHI must be password protected. You are additionally required to make every effort to protect PHI from loss due to natural causes or theft. This means you must have back-up protection for all of your records. You can do this with an external storage device, or you can use an online backup method. HIPAA requires that you have a formal Business Associate Agreement (BAA) with your online backup provider if you keep any PHI on your computer or mobile device. This means that your online backup provider gives assurance that PHI is protected, even from their own employees. The original backup provider I was using would offer a BAA with a 5-fold increase in their rates, so I shopped around and found one with secure service and a BAA for $5 per month. At the time of this writing, some good sources for HIPAA compliant online backup include carbonite.com, spideroak.com and crashplan.com. There are more, so do some comparison shopping. Also at the time of this writing, the iCloud would not sign a BAA. This means that if you have an iCloud connected to any device with PHI, the iCloud feature must be disabled from that device in order to protect PHI.[6]

You are required to keep all medical documentation for a period of time after discharge. Your state will have a medical record retention law outlining the statutory required period of time. You may see a required period of time stated in some of your network contracts; even if it isn't stated, you must comply with the statutory timeline. Your state will have special rules for the medical records of minors, usually requiring that the records be retained up to or beyond the age of majority. There is usually a requirement for notification if the records are to be destroyed. In the absence of state regulation, it is my understanding that records should be retained three years after the patient comes of age or five years after the date of discharge, whichever is longer. These records can really pile up in your home or office. Protecting them electronically is really the best way to go.

---

[6] https://www.hhs.gov/hipaa/for-professionals/special-topics/cloud-computing/index.html, June 16, 2017

Required Documents to Keep on File

Therapy Evaluation with Goals and Plan of Care

This is the foundation for providing service to your patient. This is critical and will be discussed in the next chapter.

Physician Referral

Depending upon state regulations, you may not need a physician referral before your first visit. If a physician referral is not required under state law, you may need one on file for the medical payer. Regardless of whether a payer requires it, I recommend that you get one. By routinely requesting a physician referral for all patients, I do not need to remember which insurance company requires a referral and which one does not. In addition, requesting the referral offers me an opportunity to share my plan of care with the patient's physician.

If the payer doesn't require prior authorization, I will usually write up my evaluation first and then fax it to the doctor's office, asking the Primary Care Provider (PCP) to review the evaluation and if he/she agrees with my plan of care to please fax back a referral for physical therapy services. This establishes a relationship with the PCP and helps the physician understand why I am seeing the patient and what I hope to achieve. Since many of my referrals have come from an Early Intervention agency or a family self-referral, it is good practice to let the PCP know I am seeing the patient.

If you must have a physician referral before you see the patient you will need to request the referral directly from the physician. Some physicians will request a 'physical therapy evaluation' or other professional evaluation. In that case, you will need to submit a copy of the evaluation and request a referral for your services. Other physicians will submit a 'physical therapy evaluate and treat' referral. If you receive an 'evaluate and treat' referral, once you have completed your evaluation, always fax a copy of it to the PCP with a note that says 'for your records'. This is both a courtesy and a standard means of care coordination.

If the patient ends up being a long term patient, you should perform a re-evaluation and request an updated physician referral at least annually. (I always send the physician a copy of my re-evaluation with my request for a new referral). Some payers may request a re-evaluation and physician referral more often; you usually only need a physician referral annually unless your state licensure regulations state otherwise. You will get more specific information from a payer if a prior authorization is required or if you are part of a network that has guidelines addressing this issue.

Treatment notes for each visit date

Every visit must be dated and documented. Documentation should include what you did, the length of the treatment session and your signature. You can initial each visit if your signature with your initials is at the bottom of each page. Your signature should always include your professional designation.

You do not usually need to document progress on every visit, however some s payers look for documentation that you are working on the goals established in your plan of care. A progress report can be documented intermittently, usually at least monthly. A progress report is not a re-evaluation and should not be billed as such.

When you document your treatment, keep in mind that this documentation should concur with your billing. If you bill for a service that is not documented, you have a problem. There will be more on this in the next chapter.

Required Permissions

Your patient record will need to include a signed permission to bill and permission for the payer to pay you directly. I have provided an example of my permission form in Appendix C. This is the one I am using at the printing of this manual. However, it may not meet every state's requirements for permission; you may want to use this as a guide and reword it to meet your own local requirements. If you have a long term patient, the consent signature should be updated at least annually. A payer may request that this be done more often, but I have not seen this myself.

The permission to bill requirement is part of the Form CMS -1500 which is the claim form used for all Outpatient PT, OT and SLP billing to medical service payers. There are actually two permissions which are stated as follows:

12. PATIENT'S OR AUTHORIZED PERSON'S SIGNATURE   I authorize the release of any medical or other information necessary to process this claim. I also request payment of government benefits either to myself or to the party who accepts assignment below.

13. INSURED'S OR AUTHORIZED PERSON'S SIGNATURE   I authorize payment of medical benefits to the undersigned physician or supplier for services described below.

If you have a signature that encompasses these statements on a form, you may keep this signature in the patient record. Each time you submit a bill, you state 'signature on file' for each of these statements on the Form CMS-1500.

If your patient is a long term patient, you should get a new signature at least annually. You should also get new signatures any time the patient changes insurance payers.

Signed acknowledgment of receipt of Privacy Notice

Since medical records are known to contain significant confidential information, HIPAA (Health Insurance Portability and Accountability Act) was established to impose a Federal Standard of Privacy and Security, especially for the electronic transmission, but also including all methods of sharing protected health information. I refer to HIPAA intermittently throughout this manual as a reminder of the responsibility you carry with medical service provision. Medical records need to be protected at the highest level.

The Privacy Notice describes how the patient's medical information may be used and disclosed. It also tells the patient how he/she may access this information. The notice must contain a description of the types of uses and disclosures that you, as a provider, are permitted to make for treatment, payment and healthcare operations. It must contain a description of each of the other purposes you are permitted or required to use or disclose without the patient's written consent or authorization (such as a report of child abuse). It should also include disclosures that will be made only with the patient's written authorization and that this permission may be revoked. There are other required elements of the notice and you can get specific information and more detail at *http://www.hhs.gov/ocr/privacy* a website dedicated to all things HIPAA.

Appendix D is a copy of my most recent Privacy Notice. Feel free to use it and modify it to your needs. Your professional association may have an example of one on its website. The last time I checked, the APTA (American Physical Therapy Association) provided a sample statement online. Keep in mind that I am not an attorney and that your state may have additional rules for compliance, so you may want to have an attorney review your notice and any other documents which are essential to meeting requirements of health care provision in your state.

Your patient should sign and date a statement that he/she has received a copy of the Privacy Notice. You must keep this signature on file and if your privacy policy materially changes give the patient an updated notice and obtain a new dated signature. If there is no material change in your policy notice, there is no requirement to obtain a signature of receipt more than once.

Recommended Medical Record Documentation

Summary of patient insurance policy information, including contact phone numbers

As a solo provider, you need to stay organized. Where else would you keep this information? If you have already reviewed my consent form (Appendix C), you have noticed that I have the patient insurance information and consents all on one page. This way I know I have it. If the patient insurance coverage changes, you will want a new consent for billing and payment as the participants under the covered consent will be different.

Summary of the patient's health insurance company policy requirements around your service

Whether billing multiple payers or only one payer you will want a summary of specific payer requirements in your patients' medical records. Even within one insurance company, there may be multiple plans with different rules. Some plans require prior authorization and some do not. Some plan years begin on October 1, most January 1, and there are other variations. There are wide differences in deductible amounts, copayments, allowed numbers of visits before authorization required, etc. It is just easier if you have it all written down. Appendix B is a form labeled Patient Insurance Plan Data. I created it to remind me to ask for particular information.

Just for clarification, look at the Patient Insurance Plan Data form (Appendix B). I have listed 'co-payments' and 'annual deductible' then below that I have listed 'network versus non-network'. The network versus non-network option is a reminder to determine whether you would want to pursue the option of becoming a network provider. When you call the insurance company, you can ask for copayments and deductibles for both in-network and non-network. The 'Insurance year' is the date that the annual deductible and out of pocket cost determinations begin. Sometimes an insurance plan will have a restricted number of visits per year per therapy. Sometimes the plan will have a fixed number of visits per year of PT, OT and Speech combined and sometimes the plan will combine any two of the therapies for a fixed number of visits. If you find that your therapy is combined with another for an annual number of visits, make sure the patient family understands this and works with you to determine if the patient will be receiving other therapies and how many of each the patient would need. Sometimes a payer will allow exceptions for the fixed number of visits per year per therapy, but not always. Do not count on it. You should always ask if there are predetermined restrictions around provision of your service. For instance, you may be told that the plan does not cover 'developmental delay' (to be discussed in the next chapter) or that it only covers disorders which occur as a result of an injury or illness. Some state policies do not allow these restrictions, so if you happen to know that your state policy requires insurance companies to cover birth disorders, make sure you get this clarified. State policy does not have jurisdiction over some plans, such as private payer plans or plans from other states.

Copies of all EOB's (Explanation of Benefits) and statements received for services provided to this patient.

The EOB is the statement from the healthcare payer. This document will tell you what is covered by the plan and what was paid. You must keep these documents somewhere and it only makes sense to keep them with your patient record. Larger facilities have a separate location for this, but as a solo provider, it is just easier to keep everything together. If I am keeping a patient record in a folder, I will file the EOB with the corresponding treatment notes.

Documentation of other payments received for services, including copayments and deductibles.

You need to have a record of all other payments received for the patient's services. You are required to bill for copayments and deductibles.[7] You should have some record of collecting or attempting to collect payment for this patient responsibility. If you are an Early Intervention provider, your state may have a policy that the Early Intervention Program will cover all or a portion of the patient share of reimbursement.

Also, keep in mind that the payments received from the patient (family) will need to be reported to the IRS as income. So you will need a means of keeping track of all income received.

Documentation of all correspondence and communication around this patient's services

You should keep a log of all telephone, fax, or email communications regarding this patient. Also, file other medical or educational reports which have been shared with you.

---

[7] This falls under the Federal False Claims Act, Federal Anti-Kickback Statute, and the Federal and State Insurance Fraud Laws.

Chapter 4:

Documentation

As mentioned earlier in this book, most health insurance payers are familiar with and have adopted or defer to the CMS Manual when establishing standards for service provision and this includes documentation. Because of this, even non-Medicare providers are expected to meet the standards established in those guidelines. This manual is a good resource and can be found on the Centers for Medicare and Medicaid Services website at http://www.cms.gov/. The documentation guidelines are in The Medicare Benefit Policy Manual, Chapter 15, Sections 220 and 230 and provide the minimal expectations. Some of the terminology is Medicare specific, such as 'Certification' which is the Medicare format for physician approval of the Plan of Care. Pediatric therapists would simply call this a physician referral. For that matter the 'Plan of Care' is a Medicare format that pediatric therapists would typically include as part of the evaluation or re-evaluation and treatment plan. We sometimes refer to our treatment plan as a 'plan of care', but it isn't a separate document. Overall, however, the elements of required Medicare documentation are the elements that any healthcare insurance medical necessity reviewer would expect to see in a patient's evaluation and medical file.

Keep in mind that your state or local laws or policies may require additional or slightly different documentation. These policies may be established to protect you or to re-enforce state or local practice policies. Professional guidelines of the APTA (American Physical Therapy Association), AOTA (American Occupational Therapy Association) or ASHA (American Speech-Language Hearing Association) may have additional documentation guidelines. Your professional association is also often contacted by major payers for guidance and input on policies. As far as regulatory guidelines go however, the Medicare Benefits Policy Manual is probably the most comprehensive, transparent and easily accessible resource when it comes to documentation requirements and recommendations.

The Evaluation

The evaluation is the justification for the therapy you provide. Your evaluation should be typewritten and professional in appearance. Most importantly, when it comes to billing health care insurance, your evaluation needs to demonstrate that the service you are providing is medically necessary and a condition that can and should be treated by your profession.

Those of you who have been working in hospitals or clinics may find this chapter pretty basic. But the documentation requirements for school or Early Intervention therapy are typically very different from medically based documentation requirements. In this chapter, when I speak of Early Intervention, I am referring to services provided through an IDEA Part C Early Intervention Agency.

Pediatric rehabilitation therapists who have worked primarily or more recently in schools or in Early Intervention have some preparation for writing medical evaluations. In those two settings, functionally appropriate long term goals are the standard. For instance, 'Susie will feed herself using a spoon, unassisted'. This goal is something that any reader would understand, both in content and value.

The weakness that school based or Early Intervention therapists might have is in justifying the medical necessity of the service provided. In those settings, providing support for the school staff or family may be justification enough for service, regardless of the actual needs of the child. Whereas, in the medical setting, the child is the patient and the needs of the caregiver cannot be the focus of or justification for treatment. In Early Intervention the fact of developmental delay may be the main requirement for justification of your service, whereas, a healthcare insurance payer may have a policy that says developmental delay is not a justification for service. In Schools and Early Intervention settings we are asked to be family friendly. We are required to stay positive and emphasize the child's competencies rather than his deficiencies. If you try this in the medical evaluation, your service will likely be denied payment as there is no evidence of pathology. I tell you this from experience.

In the medical evaluation, it is not enough to say the child has Down Syndrome or Cerebral Palsy and assume that services will be approved. You must identify the specific concern that you will be treating. If you simply say the child has developmental delay, your services will most assuredly be denied. If you think about it, 'developmental delay' doesn't really explain anything; it is just a general symptom. The therapist evaluation must determine and point out the specific and underlying treatable and medical pathology that may or may not be contributing to the delay and focus on that issue. Along that line, keep in mind that most medical service reviewers are not child development savvy and may not see the problem if 12 month old 'Jimmy cannot sit or crawl'. But the reviewer will recognize the problem if you say 'Jimmy lacks sufficient strength or trunk control to sit unsupported'.

Just as 'developmental delay' is a red flag term in your medical evaluation, most healthcare insurance companies additionally have a policy that 'sensory integration' is not an allowable treatment, as it is unproven. Most payers do not know what sensory integration actually is and many therapists use the term indiscriminately to cover a broad array of possible interventions. I have seen a speech therapist report stating that she would be 'addressing the patient's sensory integration concerns'. What does that mean? Payers who have a policy that does not cover sensory integration will deny the entire service, if those words are used, even if sensory concerns are not the main focus of the service. I recommend that you avoid using a single term as a broad brush to define a patient's needs. Instead, once again, you should clearly define the pathology that you have observed and plan to treat. For instance, the child may have a vestibular dysfunction, or tactile hypersensitivity. I address this topic in greater detail in Chapter 10.

In the medically based evaluation, you need to specifically point out the pathologies that you will be treating. Furthermore, these pathologies must be something that are treatable by and require the skilled services of your profession. So, you do not treat Down Syndrome, but the physical therapist does help the patient to gain strength, trunk control, endurance and the coordination required for independent mobility. The Occupational Therapist does help the patient with strength and coordination for dressing. The Speech-Language Pathologist does treat dysphagia. Your evaluation must point out the specific deficiencies that you may observe and will be treating.

What about Assessment Tools?

With regard to standardized developmental evaluations, you don't typically need them to be part of your medically oriented, discipline-specific evaluation. If a standardized developmental evaluation has already been done, you can report the findings as they support your medically oriented evaluation. But keep in mind your professional focus. So for instance, you could say that according to (Specific Test) the child was not yet functioning at a level expected for his age in when trying to eat independently. (Note I said function rather than 'development'. This is because at the time of this writing, 'developmental' is a red flag word and 'function' is a buzz word in the world of medical reimbursement). You can list the skills that he is not able to do that are related to your area of focus and that are expected of a child his age. Since the medical evaluation requires that you point out the pathologies and how these pathologies affect function, the additional standardized developmental evaluation may simply be a distraction, but you do need to know the expected age appropriate function of the child you are treating. Hopefully, as a pediatric therapist, you would be able to point out how the problem is affecting the child's expected age appropriate function.

With that said, as a pediatric rehabilitation therapist you have the knowledge and the tools to recognize and report how the pathology is affecting the expected function of children at various ages. These tools may include published assessment tools that evaluate specific aspects of child development, such as communication. That will help you determine whether the child is functioning at an age appropriate level. In fact this may help you determine that a patient does not require your services. But if, based upon your knowledge, the child is clearly functioning well below the expected level of function, you might want to use a tool to help you measure and demonstrate progress as a result of the therapy provided. Not all tools have that capability, as they will sometimes only compare the child to same aged typical children. When reporting function and in developing functional goals, you need to know that you are being realistic with regard to the child's age or capabilities. You do not always need to use a standardized developmental tool to do this. But there are other standardized tests you might use. Chapter 7 in this book will provide physical therapists and occupational therapists with additional suggestions for testing. This is your option and dependent upon your professional opinion and background.

There is most certainly a role in the medical arena for the standardized developmental assessment. The multidisciplinary developmental assessment is often one of the essential tools for helping to diagnosis certain disorders such as autism, learning disabilities, or other disorders that may sometimes be difficult to diagnose. It is also useful for helping to zero in on what areas of primary concern may exist in the child with a confusing overall picture. But remember that your specific disciplinary evaluation is to determine if this child has a specific problem that can be successfully treated by your specific profession.

Required Elements of the Evaluation

Keep in mind that this guide was written for the pediatric rehabilitation therapist who is planning to provide service as a solo practitioner. You get to determine your own policies and standards for documentation. You just need to be aware of industry standards and expectations. The following required evaluation elements are those set by the Medicare Benefits Policy Manual as described earlier in this book.

- A diagnosis. The issue of the diagnosis is sometimes the key to whether the payer will cover your service. You need to make the distinction between an overall medical diagnosis that may be related to what you are treating and the actual impairment based treatment diagnosis that is related to the service you will be providing. For instance, Muscular Dystrophy may be the medical diagnosis, but the treatment diagnosis may be 'difficulty walking'. There are ICD-10 codes that are sometimes known as condition descriptors. Currently there are ICD-10 codes for 'difficulty walking', 'abnormal gait', 'muscle weakness', 'dysphagia', 'hemiparesis', and many more. More specifics on coding will be discussed in Chapter 6. Ideally, your evaluation will include at least one medical diagnosis that is relevant to the problem you are treating, as well as your treatment diagnosis (condition descriptor). As you know, when we work with children, especially very young children, there may not yet be a medical diagnosis and that is fine, as long as you have a relevant treatment diagnosis or condition. Be aware of your state laws regarding establishing a diagnosis and stay within your scope of practice. The 'condition descriptors' are usually within the scope of practice of most therapists. Try to include all conditions and complexities that may impact your treatment.

- Objective and relevant information supporting the severity or complexity of the patient such as
    *other health services currently being provided
    *durable medical equipment such as a walker or wheelchair currently in use or needed
    *known medications
    *complicating factors such as heart or lungs, impending surgeries, or vision that may affect the pace of progress and how
    *generalized or other conditions such as junior rheumatoid arthritis, or cancer that may directly or significantly impact the rate of progress
    *known mental or cognitive disorder that will impact the rate of progress
    *other factors such as age or symptoms that may affect progress
    *previous recent therapies if known
    *general health
    *patient social support such as living with parents or in foster care or an assisted living facility
    *Documentation of measurable physical function. You can use functional assessment tools or identify functional goals which can be measured toward progress.
- Clinician's clinical judgments or subjective impressions that describe the current functional status of the condition being evaluated especially if these judgments provide further information to supplement objective measurements.
- A determination that treatment is not needed, or, if treatment is needed a prognosis for the expected outcome with a time frame and a plan of care, including goals.

There is no specification regarding the order or the format of the evaluation. This is up to you. Remember the point of the evaluation is to determine and justify whether the patient requires your service, treatment goals and plan of care.

An Example

I have included a sample of the format that I use in my evaluations in Appendix E. You can really use any format you are comfortable with, but there are specific items that should be included in every evaluation.

Child's name and date of birth
Date of the evaluation
Relevant known medical diagnoses
Treatment disorder

A short **introduction** of the patient including age, sex, reason for referral and any other essential background information.(If the child is blind and has cerebral palsy, don't forget to mention this). I have, when needed, listed all of the medical professionals currently treating the patient, as well as all of the medications the child is receiving. I also like to list any impending or past surgeries or medical treatments which may affect the outcome of my treatment.

Objective observations

You can organize your objective assessment any way you would prefer. However, remember that this is a medical evaluation and you need to look at the child from a problem focused position. Below is the way I choose to report on patients with whom I work. Speech language pathologists will sometimes use special tools and observational protocols. Occupational Therapists may find it useful to focus on different impairments, but can also use my protocol. Just try to stay as basic and concrete as you can. I pulled out all references to development and went back to the basics so that the medical reviewer could clearly see that my evaluation was a physical therapy evaluation and not a developmental evaluation. My observations are listed as follows:

Observations and testing:

Strength, motor control and endurance You don't have to do muscle testing, but you can sometimes observe whether a child has 2/5 versus 4/5 strength in certain muscle groups. You can describe activities which demonstrate muscle weakness. You might say 'Jason lacks sufficient strength in his shoulders for supporting himself on hands and knees.' Or you can report endurance by saying 'Tess lies down to rest every 3 feet when crawling'.

Joint mobility/stability: You can report specific joint tightness or hypermobility or just say WNL (a common abbreviation for 'within normal limits')

Skills: Report what the patient is doing and not yet doing. This is where you use your knowledge on child development and point out what activities this child is not yet doing that he should be able to do. I always start with listing a few key present activities and end with what is missing.

Assessment: If you haven't yet noticed, I have followed the SOAP (Subjective, Objective, Assessment, Plan) format for my evaluation. But with regard to the 'Assessment' I have two sections as follows:

Summary of concerns and potential for improvement: Give an overview of what you believe is the primary problem(s) you will be treating. This is also the place where you will say that the child's vision impairment or recent surgery or other issues may complicate your treatment approach or slow the progress you might typically expect. Then give an honest assessment of what you believe the child's potential for improvement would be.

Goals: You need short term and long term goals. You want to be able to demonstrate progress over the short term, but also give the reader a clear picture of where you are going, or what success will look like. I also list the date the goal was established.

Plan: The typical payer would like to know your planned frequency and criteria for discharge. This is modeled after the Medicare policy manual. If you determine that treatment is not required, you may say something like 'evaluation has determined that this patient does not require the specialized skills of a physical therapist at this time'. You may also recommend evaluation by another profession.

Be as specific as you can reasonably be. I prefer to give myself a little flexibility in my plan. So I may say 'Daniel will benefit from physical therapy one to two times a week with caregiver follow through on recommended activities'. My 'criteria for discharge' is usually something such as 'when goals are met and as agreed upon by family and physician.' Some payers may want a specific timeline. If you have already pointed out that there may be complicating factors, they will usually work with you if you surpass your predicted timeline.

The Re-evaluation

The re-evaluation is not just a progress report or reassessment. You cannot bill a progress report or reassessment as a re-evaluation. The focus of the re-evaluation should be an evaluation of progress toward current goals, making a professional judgment about continued care, retesting areas that should be tested, modifying goals and/or treatment or terminating services. In the past, the re-evaluation code has been misunderstood by therapists and overused. So some payers have begun to deny payment for any re-evaluations. If this happens, submit a copy of your re-evaluation for review.

The re-evaluation requires the same professional skills as an evaluation. Your re-evaluation holds the same weight as an evaluation and so you do not need to do a re-evaluation unless requested or unless the patient's condition has changed significantly, there are new clinical findings, or if the patient is not responding to therapy. Intermittently, the payer may ask for a re-evaluation, especially if one is needed for authorization of continued services. Always write up your re-evaluation as a formal document, just as you would an evaluation.

I typically use the same format for my re-evaluation as I use for my evaluation. My introduction states how much therapy the patient has received and if there have been gaps in service due to illness or surgery. I report on the same areas I reported on in the evaluation. I additionally list which goals have been met and may add a goal or two, if my patient is progressing well. This will be your opportunity to adjust and justify a change in your plan of care if needed.

Progress Report

Medicare and thus most Healthcare Insurance payers expect to see intermittent progress reports throughout the duration of treatment. This is not reimbursed separately. At this time, Medicare requires a progress report at least once during each 30 calendar days or at least once every 10 treatment days, whichever is less. Most insurance payers aren't so specific. The progress report is less formal and so can be hand-written or typed as a part of the treatment note.

Some therapists write a progress report for every treatment session. Treatment notes are required for every treatment session. You do not have to report on progress for every session. Many therapists have traditionally called their treatment notes 'progress notes' and so there is confusion regarding a progress report, a progress note and a treatment note.

The CMS Manual does not use the term 'progress note'. You will often find that healthcare insurance payers will request progress reports and treatment notes to help to determine the medical necessity of your service.

I typically write a progress report once a month and my treatment notes are separately written for each treatment date. If you write a progress note for every session that includes progress and treatment provided, that's fine. If you do this, you do not have to write a separate progress report. Make sure your progress report addresses at least one of the goals that have been established as a part of your treatment plan.

If you have worked in a hospital setting or a large facility, you may have been required to follow a stricter or slightly different protocol. Different settings such as hospitals, home health care agencies or other settings have slightly different rules for documentation. In many cases, these large facility policies are an attempt to meet the documentation requirements of all settings served by the facility. Remember, this particular guide is for the solo practitioner who provides outpatient pediatric physical rehabilitation.

Treatment Note

There must be a treatment note for each treatment session. Here are the required elements of a treatment note:

> Date of Service
> Service provided
> Treatment time
> Signature and credentials of provider

Some specific requirements are dependent upon the types of treatment codes you may use for billing. Codes will be discussed in more detail in another chapter, but for treatment documentation, you need to remember that there are timed codes and untimed codes.

Timed codes are those codes that are billed according to how much time is spent with the patient. These codes are typically billed in 15 minute increments. Putting it simply, a 30 minute visit would require 2 units of the code billed. Most Pediatric Physical Therapists and Occupational Therapists provide treatments that are billed in timed codes. Sometimes Speech Language Pathologist (SLP) will provide a timed code session, such as cognitive training. SLPs must remember that they are not allowed to combine timed code services in the same session as the untimed 'speech therapy' code service.[8]

The Speech Therapy untimed codes are billed on a per visit basis. This means that one unit equals one visit regardless of the amount of time spent providing the service. Reimbursement is based upon the expected cost of providing the service. Most Speech Language Pathologists typically provide treatments that are billed in untimed codes. SLPs can bill for an evaluation and treatment in one session, so with this exception, 1 unit for an evaluation and 1 unit for treatment would be billed for one session. These are two separate and distinct procedures.

It is possible for physical therapists and occupational therapists to have a treatment session that includes both timed and untimed codes in one session. For instance, the Physical Therapist may provide an evaluation (untimed code) and treatment (timed code) in one session. When this happens,, the amount of time spent for evaluation and the amount of time spent for treatment must be documented separately.

The CPT code book has descriptors of the codes, including whether they are timed or untimed.

When you document your treatment session, your treatment note should support the codes you have billed. If you bill the code for Neuromuscular Re-education, 97112, then your treatment notes should say you provided at least some of the service included in the descriptor for that code, such as balance and posture activities. If you additionally billed another treatment code such as 97110, therapeutic exercise, your documentation should include words that are part of the CPT code book descriptor for that service, such as strength and endurance.

You also must include the amount of time spent providing the treatment. This is important. If your treatment notes are audited, the auditor must be able to verify that your treatment documentation supports what you billed. If your entire session was spent providing service that falls under timed treatment, then you only need to include the total time of your treatment session. However, if you treatment session includes both timed and untimed codes, then you should include two times. Document the total time of the session and the time spent providing timed code service. So if the Occupational Therapist provided an evaluation and treatment in one

---

[8]   CHAP 11.doc,Version 16.3,CHAPTER XI,MEDICINE,EVALUATION AND MANAGEMENT SERVICES,CPT CODES 90000 – 99999 FOR NATIONAL CORRECT CODING INITIATIVE POLICY MANUAL FOR MEDICARE SERVICES

session her notes might include: Total time of session—1 hour, timed treatment—30 minutes. Or it could be documented as evaluation 35 minutes, treatment 25 minutes.

Requirements for documentation of time have changed over the years. This is something you should check out intermittently on the CMS website at http://www.cms.gov/. For instance, a few years ago, there was an expectation that the amount of time spent for each treatment code should be documented. However, this rule often lead to incorrect billing and so now the rule is that the total amount of time spent on timed treatments should be documented. See 'Rule of 8' in Chapter 6 in this book. I have also been asked if the therapist must document the time of day the session started and ended. I have not seen this requirement on any regulation that applies to outpatient therapy services. I have never documented time of day of the session and have never been refused payment when my notes have been reviewed. If you work in a setting that has the possibility of providing more than one treatment session in one day, such as a hospital setting, it is logical that you would need to supply this information in order to demonstrate that more than one session was provided. Once again, policies can change; check out requirements on the CMS website intermittently.

Remember that the treatment note does not have to include a progress report, but there is certainly no rule against it. I try not to get too wordy in my treatment notes, so that they are not burdensome. I might occasionally write a simple statement such as 'Joey took two steps unsupported', just to document critical milestone achievements. Mostly I just say what I did.

There are no specific rules around the format to be used for treatment notes. I used to just write a narrative on two or three lines, including the date and time and followed with my signature. Most therapists are familiar with this format. However, when I owned my multidisciplinary company with almost 30 therapists, I found that I needed to create a form that insured that the therapists remembered to include all of the elements required in the treatment note. I learned of a format being used by a nearby hospital and modified it for my own use. I have also used this form as a solo provider for several reasons. One reason is that it has boxes in which I need to fit my notes and this makes me stay brief. The other reason is that it allows me to address each treatment goal with my treatment notes providing an ongoing reminder of my treatment plan. This form is on Appendix F. I realize it is a little unconventional, but I have submitted it for records reviews when requested and no one seems to mind it. I have also attached another format (Appendix G) which I have been using more recently. This format allows me to complete one document each month, so I have separate blocks for treatment notes, a list of my goals and progress toward goals and a place to write up a monthly summary and parent participation.

A note to Speech Language Pathologists, although the typical coding for your services are untimed codes, you should still include the amount of time spent in treatment. If you are providing two different services in one session, such as Speech Therapy and Feeding and Swallowing therapy, I would break it down and document how much time was spent providing each service. When you provide two different services, you can certainly document those services separately and on different forms. If you choose to document on the same form, you must be careful to insure that documentation reflects separate treatments as well as progress toward goals in both arenas.

Your signature and professional designation are required documentation to the treatment note. If you have several treatment sessions documented on one page, you may initial each note and then sign the bottom of the page with your professional designation. For clarification it would be appropriate to additionally add your initials on the bottom of the page, after your signature and professional designation.

There are slightly different documentation rules for qualified assistants and their supervisors. This guide was written for the solo practitioner, but if you additionally use the services of an assistant, you should refer to the CMS Manual [Chapter] 220.3 E. for specific information. Your state regulations may have additional regulations. Please note that there was no reference to assistant documentation for evaluations and re-evaluations because this is not allowed. Additionally, keep in mind, your state regulations may not allow the services of an assistant in the patient home setting unless you meet additional licensure requirements. Some payers do not reimburse the services of an assistant for outpatient therapy in any setting, although progress is being made toward policy changes. Check on the policies of your payer before your assistant provides outpatient therapy services.

Discharge Note

The discharge note is simply an explanation of why services were discontinued. It may be included in a re-evaluation that was performed and determined that services were no longer required.

The discharge note may also simply be included in a treatment note. You may document the treatment provided, say that goals have been met and that your services have been discontinued. If this is the case, I will often summarize how the goals have been met and that physical therapy services are no longer required at this time. Technically, if you just say 'the goals have been met' that is explanation enough.

Sometimes therapy is discontinued for unrelated reasons. The discharge note may be written separate from other documentation. Let me give you some examples of discharge notes I have written.

"Patient and family have moved away from the area. He should resume physical therapy services in his new location.'

'Patient deceased'

'Patient family is experiencing unrelated stresses and has requested a break from physical therapy. It would be appropriate to resume services in the future when they are ready.'

'Patient had surgery and is unable to participate in physical therapy. The patient should be able to resume physical therapy in the future, but we will need a physician referral with post-surgery precautions from the surgeon at that time.' (In Colorado, we are able to see patients without a physician referral. However, it would be prudent to make sure the surgeon is in agreement with the resumption of physical therapy).

Change of service providers

Sometimes circumstances require that the patient must change providers for the same service. If the service provider change is within the same company or agency, the payer is unconcerned, as there is no change in billing or service authorizations. However, this would not be the case for a solo practitioner. If there is a need to change providers, the payer will sometimes request documentation from the previous provider. This is to insure that there is no duplication of services and that there has been coordination of care between the two providers.

Examples of change of service provider documentation may be as follows:

'Family is unable to keep scheduled appointments. They have switched to a provider who is better able to meet their scheduling needs. Documentation of prior services has been shared with the new provider as requested by the family.'

'Patient physical therapy service needs are unable to be met in his home at this time. Services will be switched to the clinic environment. Current physical therapy documentation will be shared with the new provider and with parent permission.'

Chapter 5:

Billing for Outpatient Pediatric Rehabilitation Services

The Claim Form

Methods of Billing

Outpatient Pediatric physical therapy, occupational therapy and speech language pathology services are billed on Form CMS-1500. Many health insurance payers provide online access to their forms allowing you to use the payer website to bill that payer electronically, free of charge. Additionally, there are websites which allow you to bill any or most payers electronically using only one system. Some of these web-based electronic billing companies charge a small monthly fee. Office Ally can be accessed at www.officeally.com and offers free CMS-1500 electronic transmission. Sometimes your reimbursement is faster if you use the payer's website, but each website is slightly different, so if your patients are covered by multiple payers, it may be easier to use just one electronic billing website such as Office Ally.

It is important to know that you DO NOT need to invest in an expensive electronic documentation and billing system in order to see patients and bill electronically. Those systems are designed for groups with multiple providers and large numbers of patients, allowing for a more streamlined and simplified process. It would not be cost effective for a solo practitioner with a small caseload to invest in a system such as this. The large-scale electronic billing system could be right for you if your plans include significant growth and expansion.

Another option includes paying someone to do your medical billing. However, this does not let you off the hook for understanding the proper use of medical billing codes and obtaining required signatures and documentation. The paid medical biller simply inputs the codes and dates of services you have designated. The paid medical biller is not your office assistant and you cannot expect that person to obtain signatures or maintain your medical records. You will see that medical billing is the easiest part of the whole process. Once you have done the work of providing the service, obtaining the required signatures and information, and accumulating the required documentation, it makes little sense to pay someone to do something that takes less than one minute per date of service. I have also taught my office assistants how to bill for services as my practice grew. Formal medical billing training is not a requirement.

You do not have to bill electronically. The Form CMS-1500 is a paper form which can be purchased directly from the US Government Printing Office, or easiest of all, you can purchase a downloadable form online in a Word or Excel format and keep it on your desktop. I recently downloaded a PDF document onto my desktop for free. All payers will accept the paper bill and some actually will only accept paper bills attached to required documentation for all outpatient therapy services. For instance, I bill all of my patient services electronically except for one. This patient's insurance requires a copy of my evaluation, the doctor referral and my respective treatment notes along with the paper Form CMS-1500 every time I bill. The nice thing about the downloadable form is that you can pre-populate all of the patient information and save it to your desktop, then each month you only have to fill in the treatment dates, codes, amounts and totals, print it, sign it and mail it. I purchased my form from www.MedicalFormSoftware.com and it is currently available for $99.00, but you may find a better deal from another company. If you want more specific information on the form itself, go to http://www.cms.gov/ElectronicBillingEDITrans/16_1500.asp .

Completing the Form CMS-1500

The Form CMS-1500 is a universal billing form and you will see that it is meant to be used for a variety of services. If you bill electronically, regardless of the online format, the resulting product is the Form CMS-1500. Once you understand how to use the paper format of the form, all of the electronic formats you run across will make sense and you will understand what is required when you fill in the blanks. You will find a copy of the Form CMS-1500 in Appendix H.   In this section of the chapter I will refer to the box numbers so you can find them on the paper form representation. However, some electronic formats do not look like the form and do not have the box numbers included. Instead they are just verbally labeled, but the result is the same.

If you want detailed and precise instructions for the completion of this form, you can download the 64 page guide to your desktop. This gives details that are mostly obvious within the form. Go to http://nucc.org/

The following is a summary of what the pediatric physical therapist, occupational therapist or speech-language pathologist needs to know to correctly complete the form. Don't be afraid. Once you populate the patient and carrier information on the electronic version or the paper version of the form, you will not have to do it again, unless the payer information changes. If you happen to use the payer website, you will not need to complete that information as it will already be in the system.

Carrier Information

At the top right side of the form is a blank space for the carrier information. The carrier is the payer or administrator who handles the claim. On the paper form, you would include the information found on the patient's insurance card typically stating 'Submit claims to:' a recipient and address. If you are billing electronically, the website will include a drop down with the electronic billing codes associated with the payer.

Patient and Insured Information (Boxes 1 through 11)

Completion of this section is mostly self-explanatory. Make certain to have the correct 'Insured's ID number', or Medical Identification number. This number must match the patient or insured's name and date of birth. If this information is not correct, the claim will be denied as 'patient is not a covered beneficiary'.

In the case of working with children, you will usually need to include both the patient information and the insured information. The insured is the person who holds the policy, usually a parent who is covered by an employee health plan. You should have gathered all of this information when you obtained permission to bill. Sometimes the patient is the insured, for instance, the child has Medicaid or Child Health Plan (CHP) coverage and the parent is not on the plan. If the patient is the insured, then you do not have to duplicate your information in the 'insured' section. If the patient has two insurance sources (not including Medicaid), for instance if each parent has a health care plan that includes the child, then the 'other insured' information should be included.

The address is the patient's permanent address, not a school, grandmother's house or any other possible location where the patient may temporarily be staying.

If the patient condition is due to an employment injury (not likely for children) or an accident that may be the subject of a lawsuit, the payer may withhold payment until it is determined whether another source may cover the service. It is possible that the payer will cover the service and seek remuneration from the other source. Regardless, you should answer the questions in Box 10 honestly.

If the child has Medicaid as well as private healthcare insurance, Medicaid is always the payer of last resort. When billing the primary payer, you do not list Medicaid as another health benefit. This would alert the payer that costs may be shared with another health insurance plan and this is not the case. When billing Medicaid, you would, however, list the private healthcare insurance as another health benefit plan and complete Section 9 with 'other insured' information. If you are billing Medicaid to attempt to recover copayment or deductible costs relative to the primary payer, then you would necessarily include the amount already paid by the primary payer in Box 29 ('amount paid').

Patient or Authorized Person's Signatures

You do not have to have the patient or parent sign the form every time you submit a bill. However, do not take this section lightly. You are required to get these signatures. Once you have these signatures you can keep them on file. Most payers do not specify how frequently you are required to get these signatures. Usually, the signature will cover the episode of care. You may have the patient sign a statement which says the authorization applies to all occasions of services until it is revoked. However, some payers may require an annual update. In cases where you may see the patient over a long period of time, even if only intermittently, then you should update these signatures at least annually.

Do not bill for services until you have these signatures. You may ask the patient to sign a statement that includes information from both Boxes 12 and 13 and that is fine. I have included a sample statement in Appendix C. Make sure the patient dates the signature. If you do not want to create a separate document, you can always ask the patient to sign an incomplete CMS-1500 with the patient information included, and keep that on file.

Box 12 says
READ BACK OF FORM BEFORE COMPLETING AND SIGNING THIS FORM
12. PATIENT'S OR AUTHORIZED PERSON'S SIGNATURE   I authorize the release of any medical or other information necessary to process this claim. I also request payment of government benefits either to myself or to the party who accepts assignment below.

SIGNED _____signature on file_____   DATE _____give date of signature_____

You can state 'signature on file' or 'SOF' on the signature line if you have the signed document in the patient record. This document must be kept with the patient record and ready to submit for proof of signature at any time, including after the patient is discharged from service.

There are several items of information on the back of the Form CMS-1500. The back of the form explains in greater detail how this information may be used and what type of information may be used to process the claim. This information is typically also included on your patient privacy statement that is provided to the patient to meet HIPAA standards. In addition it states that it is mandatory for the patient to tell the payer if the patient knows another party is responsible for paying for the treatment. This is particularly important for the parent of a child with healthcare insurance and Medicaid to understand. Medicaid should not be billed until other payers have been given the opportunity to pay.

Box 13 says
13. INSURED'S OR AUTHORIZED PERSON'S SIGNATURE   I authorize payment of medical benefits to the undersigned physician or supplier for services described below.   SIGNED _____ signature on file _____

This signature authorizes the payer to pay you directly. This should be signed if you expect direct payment. If this is not signed, payment will go to the patient. This would be appropriate if the patient paid the full cost of the service to you in advance. Otherwise, if the payment goes to the patient, you will need to bill the patient for the amount as well. You may keep a single signature on file in the patient records.

Physician or Supplier Information

I typically leave Boxes 14 through 20 blank. The payers I work with do not require them and most of the information is not relevant to pediatric patients. Most non-Medicare payers, including state Medicaid programs, do not require you to list the name of the referring provider as requested in Box 17, so you can leave that blank as well. If requested, you can supply it later and that will cue you to provide it for future submissions. If you are seeing a Medicare patient, the referring physician information is required.

Box 21 is crucial.

This box allows you to list up to four diagnoses. The diagnoses are indicated by ICD-10 codes. I will go into detail with regard to the process of selecting the correct ICD-10 code later in the next chapter. You are only to list the diagnosis or diagnoses you are treating during your billed sessions in this box. You should not list every possible diagnosis the patient has. You only list the conditions your treatments are addressing. Many therapists who work with children get this wrong. If the treatment you provide does not correctly match the diagnosis listed, you will not be paid. So if you are providing speech therapy to a child with cancer and you list cancer as the diagnosis you are treating, then your payment will be denied. NEWS FLASH! SPEECH THERAPY DOES NOT CURE CANCER! This is an obvious example of a diagnosis that is irrelevant to the condition being treated. Instead, the speech therapist may actually be treating 'cognitive communication deficit' which is ICD-10 code R41.841 or 'oral stage dysphagia' which is ICD-10 code R13.11. Some examples are less obvious but just as important to realize. For example the occupational therapist should not list muscular dystrophy as the condition being treated. Even though the muscular dystrophy likely contributed to the condition you are treating, you must specifically state (to the extent coding allows) the condition being treated. For example, you may list ICD-10 code M62.9 for muscle disorder.

If you look ahead to Box 24 E. you will see a column for 'DIAGNOSIS POINTER'. On each line, you will match the treatment procedure being billed (by listing the letter you have assigned to your diagnosis code) with the diagnosis or diagnoses that procedure addressed. The procedure code on that line in Column D must be an allowable procedure for the diagnosis or diagnoses listed in Column E. This will be the key to successful medical billing. It is possible that you may have been lucky in the past and your state Medicaid program may even allow you to use Down Syndrome as a diagnosis for your treatment. This would be an example of incorrect coding for PT, OT and SLP services; most healthcare insurance payers expect you to be more specific.

Box 22 only applies to resubmission of claims (or corrected claims) and appears to only relate to Medicaid claims. Private payers are not usually tuned in to this box. If I need to submit a corrected claim to a healthcare payer, I will print in large letters 'CORRECTED CLAIM' across the top. Most payers want your corrected claims to be submitted on paper, with copies of treatment notes and reports, so they can verify that your correction is legitimate. Some payers allow you to submit a corrected claim online and will have a box that allows you to designate it as a corrected claim.

Box 23 is self-explanatory. If you are required to have prior authorization for your services, the payer likely assigned a number to that prior authorization. You will find the number on the letter or form you received. If you are billing on the payer's website the authorization number may already be in their system.

Box 24 A is DATE(S) OF SERVICE. Each service provided requires its own line. For outpatient rehabilitation, each date of service requires its own line as well. Even though the date includes a FROM and TO category, do not try to group several sessions on one line. There are specific rules around grouping services on one line and they do not apply to our services. Since you are billing one service on one date per line, you do not have to complete the 'TO' column. However, some online programs require both 'FROM' and 'TO' to be completed, so you would provide the same date in each category. Completing both date categories presents more opportunities to make mistakes, so check your work. Let me tell you from experience, it takes a lot more time to go back and correct a mistake that has been submitted, than it does to get it right the first time. Making clerical errors delays payment significantly, sometimes by months.

Box 24 B is 'Place of Service'. You must include this category. Service locations have been assigned a 2 digit code. If you are providing services in the patient's natural environments, then most natural environments would be categorized under 12 (HOME). If you are renting or if you own the service location, then that is your office (11). Below are listed some codes for places of service which might be covered by solo practitioner pediatric outpatient rehabilitation therapists.

02---telehealth (the location where health services and health related services are provided or received, through telecommunications technology). Make sure you meet state requirements or your professional organization's requirements for provision of telehealth before providing this service

03—School (a facility whose primary purpose is education)

04—Homeless shelter (a facility or location whose primary purpose is to provide temporary housing to homeless individuals)

11—Office (Location other than a hospital, skilled nursing facility, military treatment facility, community health center, state or local public health clinic, or intermediate care facility, where the health professional routinely provides health examination, diagnosis, and treatment of illness or injury on an ambulatory basis.)

12—Home (A location other than a hospital or other facility, where the patient receives care in a private residence.)

14—Group Home (A residence with shared living areas, where clients receive supervision and other services such as social and/or behavioral services, custodial service, and minimal services.)

A foster home is designated as a 'home' for children. If you are paying rent for any space in which you are providing service, then that location can be designated as 'office'. More detailed information and more codes can be found at http://www.cms.gov/manuals/downloads/clm104c26.pdf . See section 10.5 on that document.

Box 24 C is an 'emergency' indicator and does not apply to outpatient pediatric rehabilitation services.

Box 24 D is the area for you to list the CPT code that describes the service you provided. Pediatric physical therapists and occupational therapists typically provide a small range of services which are billed under timed codes in 15 minute increments. The majority of services provided by pediatric SLPs are billed with untimed codes. I will discuss the specifics of measuring your time and assigning codes to your work later in this chapter. Your CPT codes are billed in units as defined in the CPT coding manual. Modifiers are rarely used, so we will discuss them later in the chapter. For now, let's just look at completing the form.

24 A. Dates of service	B. LOCATION OF SERVICE	C. EMG	D. PROCEDURES, SERVICES OR SUPPLIES	E. DIAGNOSIS POINTER	F. CHARGES	G. DAYS or UNITS	H. EPSDT	I. ID QUAL	J. PROVIDER ID RENDERING
11/01/2017	12		97110	A	160.00	4		NPI	9999999999
11/08/2017	12		97110	A	120.00	3		NPI	9999999999
11/08/2017	12		97112	A	40.00	1		NPI	9999999999

Above I have presented an example of billing and coding information for two dates of service, using timed codes. The reason I am presenting an example is to demonstrate how you should break down your charges. Assuming the physical therapist has determined that her timed treatment procedures would be billed at $40.00 per 15 minute unit, you can see that her charges on each line reflect the full amount of the charge for the units being billed on that line. On both dates, she worked directly with the patient for one hour. However, on 11/08/2017 she provided two different treatment procedures. She had to bill each procedure separately on its respective date of service. The total amount billed for each date remains the same.

24 A. Dates of service	B. LOCATION OF SERVICE	C. EMG	D. PROCEDURES, SERVICES OR SUPPLIES	E. DIAGNOSIS POINTER	F. CHARGES	G. DAYS or UNITS	H. EPSDT	I. ID QUAL	J. PROVIDER ID RENDERING
11/01/2017	12		92507	A	80.00	1		NPI	9999999999
11/08/2017	12		92507	A	80.00	1		NPI	9999999999
11/08/2017	12		92526	B	70.00	1		NPI	9999999999

The above example reflects billing and coding information provided for two dates of service, using untimed codes for Speech Therapy. The SLP provided speech therapy on 11/01/2017. However on 11/08/2017 she provided speech therapy and treatment of swallowing dysfunction. Each of these codes is untimed and reimbursement rates are fixed, regardless of the time spent during treatment. Please note that the diagnosis pointer would necessarily be different for the swallowing dysfunction procedure than it would be for the speech therapy procedure. In this example the speech therapy treatment would be for a speech related disorder and the swallowing therapy would be for a swallowing disorder.

As you can see the relationship between Boxes 24 D, E, F and G are crucial elements in reimbursement. You need to get this right.

A little more information on Box 24 E (DIAGNOSIS POINTER). You may just be using one diagnosis or condition descriptor to reflect the reason for your service provision. However, you may list up to four diagnosis codes in Box 21. The diagnosis pointer is the number you have assigned to the diagnosis listed in Box 21. When listing your procedure code, the first diagnosis pointer listed should be the primary diagnosis you were treating using that procedure. If you were additionally treating other diagnoses, you may add them in the same box, in order of priority. Do not use commas. You should never list the actual ICD-10 code in Box 24 E.

Document your charges in Box 24 F. Decide in advance how much you will charge for each service code. Remember that the amount in Box F should reflect the number of units you are billing for that particular code on that line. The same rate must be charge for all payers, even though each payer will not reimburse at the same rate. You do not need to have the same charges for each code.

Box 24 H refers to EPSTDT (Early & Periodic Screening, Diagnosis and Treatment) related services under Medicaid. Sometimes pediatric PT, OT or SLP services will be provided under that specific designation. If this is the case, you will know it. Otherwise, mark N for no, or leave it blank.

Boxes 24 I and J refer to the NPI number. As a solo practitioner pediatric physical rehabilitation therapist you should have an NPI number. Details regarding obtaining an NPI number are discussed in the first chapter.

Box 25. FEDERAL TAX I.D. NUMBER is the number of the billing provider listed in Box 33 (you). You can use your social security number or an EIN (Employer Identification Number). Understand that this number will be used for tax reporting purposes. The number should match with the person or entity listed in Box 33. If you are billing on the payer website, the payer likely already has this information and you will not need to repeat it.

Box 26. PATIENT'S ACCOUNT NO is any method you choose to identify your patient. I usually use first name initial and last name in all capitals.

Box 27. ACCEPT ASSIGNMENT? is asking whether you agree to accept the total reimbursement allowed by the payer as full payment. You are not agreeing to accept what the payer pays as payment in full. The 'allowed' payment is the reimbursement amount that the payer has determined you should be paid once all payments are received. This amount is the total you will receive once copayments, deductibles and health insurance payments are received. Most network provider contracts require that you accept assignment.

Box 28 is your total charge for all of the services and dates listed (the total of all charges listed in Column 24 F.

Box 29 is any amount already paid by the client and/or other payers for that service. If you did not collect the patient copayment in advance, you may leave it blank or put a zero in the box.

Box 31 includes your signature, credentials and the date signed. This is not included on the electronic format, but this information is already on file with the web-based billing format you may use. Please understand what you are signing. By signing this form or submitting it electronically, you are certifying that you agree to everything on the back of Form CMS-1500 and that you are a qualified provider. You are saying that you provided the services as billed. You are agreeing to follow all of the rules and regulations around the billing and provision of your services. Furthermore, you are saying that you understand that any false claims, statement, or documents, or concealment of a material fact, may be prosecuted under applicable Federal or State laws.

Box 32 requires the address of the location of service provision, unless service was provided in the patient's home, then you will leave that box blank. You do not need to use commas, periods or other punctuation. Box 32a is the NPI number of the location. If the electronic version won't allow this information, just leave it blank.

Box 33 is for your name (or your company name) and address, as well as your contact phone number. This is where you want payment to go. You must include this information for payment. Box 33 a. is for your NPI number, but I usually leave it blank. Again, if you a billing online, this information is already in the system.

So that's it. You now know how to complete the form for billing. Once you understand what the form is asking of you, you can see that the important part is to understand what codes are appropriate for your services, as well as rules around the actual provision of your services.

SO FAR

On your first visit with the patient, you gave the parent a copy of your privacy statement and requested signatures which verify receipt of that statement, permission to share information required for billing, and permission for the payer to reimburse you directly for services provided. You gathered the patient's billing information including primary and secondary payers. You requested authorization for your services, if needed. You have all of this information in a patient file, as well as your evaluation which includes goals and a treatment plan. You additionally have properly documented treatment notes for each session.

You really are ready to submit bills for your services.

CODING RULES

It is one thing to fill out the form and fill in the blanks. You submit the bill and get paid and everything is good. Right? Well, it really can be that easy, as long as you know what you are doing. Coding rules abound and if you get it wrong, you may be asked to return some money. It is best to get it right in the first place.

There are two types of reviews you may experience as a solo practitioner. One is a medical necessity review. This usually happens before payment occurs, but can happen at any point during your episode of care. The payer wants to have a look at your medical records (your evaluation and treatment notes as well as any relevant referrals) to see if your service is a service that is covered by the payer. This is where all of the good medically oriented documentation discussed in the previous chapter comes in to play. If your records meet the payer's requirements for medically necessary service provision, then all is well.

There is another type of review. This is usually referred to as a payer audit. This occurs after payment has been made. Sometimes, for example, the audit determines that the payer made a mistake. Maybe the payer incorrectly classified you as a network provider when you were really a non-network provider. This may mean that the payer paid too great of a share of the bill, wants their money back and you need to bill the patient for the difference. There are other similar mistakes the payer can make.

Most often, when the payer is doing an audit of your records, the payer wants to know if you billed correctly. The payer wants to look at your treatment notes and match what you said you did to your bill. This will typically only happen if the payer observes unusual billing patterns or if a patient complains that he did not receive treatment that was billed.

You can have peace of mind if you understand the rules around use of the codes and if your documentation supports your billing.

In some situations you won't be paid in the first place if you incorrectly code your bill. This most often happens if the diagnosis code is wrong. So let's start there, in the next chapter.

Chapter 6:

Coding for Diagnoses and Services

ICD 10 Codes
(The International Classification of Diseases, 10th Revision)

As pediatric therapists who work in multiple settings, the rules for justification for services can be confounding. For Instance, in order to qualify for Early Intervention services, a diagnosis of Down Syndrome is justification enough for services. Also, in the school setting, a child with Down Syndrome will automatically qualify for Special Education, but not necessarily need your specific therapy. When it comes to billing Health Care Insurance companies, the diagnosis of Down Syndrome is not a factor. In fact, in many cases, if you list Down Syndrome as the treatment diagnosis, you will be denied payment. The Health Insurance payer wants to know specifically what you are doing with this child. Why does this child need your service?

Here is a description distinguishing the difference between a medical diagnosis and a treatment diagnosis provided in the CMS Manual from the Centers for Medicaid and Medicare website:

Evaluation shall include:

A diagnosis (where allowed by state and local law) and description of the specific problem(s) to be evaluated and/or treated. The diagnosis should be specific and as relevant to the problem to be treated as possible. In many cases, both a medical diagnosis (obtained from a physician/NPP) and an impairment based treatment diagnosis related to treatment are relevant. The treatment diagnosis may or may not be identified by the therapist, depending on their scope of practice. Where a diagnosis is not allowed, use a condition description similar to the appropriate ICD code. For example the medical diagnosis made by the physician is CVA; however, the treatment diagnosis or condition description for PT may be abnormality of gait, for OT, it may be hemiparesis, and for SLP, it may be dysphagia. For PT and OT, be sure to include the body part evaluated. Include all conditions and complexities that may impact the treatment. A description might include, for example, the premorbid function, date of onset, and current function;

Just so you are clear, a 'condition descriptor' is an ICD-10 code which describes a condition which the therapist (or other medical professional) is trained to identify and can therefore label. A medical diagnosis is a diagnosis which requires the physician evaluation and related medical tests to determine the diagnosis conclusively. So, Muscular Dystrophy and Down Syndrome require specific medical tests which can only be ordered by a physician and therefore can only be diagnosed by a physician. Muscle weakness can be determined by the physical therapist or the occupational therapist within their scope of practice. If the physician refers to you a patient with Down Syndrome, your evaluation will determine what condition your are treating and you will then list that condition on your bill.

It is helpful to become familiar with your options for ICD-10 coding. This is not a perfect system, but it is what we have to work with. Just keep in mind that it is not appropriate to use a general medical diagnosis.

You have free access to ICD-10 codes online. Just run a search on 'ICD-10 Codes' and many sites will pop up. My current favorite is http://www.icd10data.com. I am comfortable with its navigation system, but you may find another website that suits your style of navigation. It helps to know what you are looking for. Below are some examples of ICD-10 codes that might be used by pediatric physical therapists and occupational therapists. Note that these are 'condition descriptors' and as therapists you can use these codes in the 'Diagnosis' section of the billing form.

G80.0	Spastic quadriplegic cerebral palsy
G80.1	Spastic diplegic cerebral palsy
G80.3	Athetoid cerebral palsy, dyskinetic cerebral palsy
G80.4	Ataxic cerebral palsy
G82.20	Paralysis of lower trunk and legs
G82.22	Paraplegia, paralysis of legs, incomplete
M62.81	Muscle weakness (generalized)
M62.9	Disorder of muscle, unspecified
Q66.5	Congenital pes planus, flat foot
Q66.6	In-toeing, other congenital valgus deformities of feet
Q68.0	Congenital torticollis
R25.1	Tremor, unspecified
R25.8	Other abnormal involuntary movements (includes athetosis, clonus, dystonia)
R26.0	Ataxic gait, staggering gait
R26.1	Paralytic gait, Spastic gait
R26.2	Difficulty in walking
R26.89	Other abnormalities of gait and mobility
R27.0	Ataxia, unspecified
R29.3	Abnormal posture
R29.818	Other symptoms and signs involving the nervous system
R48.2	Apraxia
R62.51	Failure to thrive, Failure to gain weight
R63.3	Feeding difficulties

The above list is just a sample of possibilities for PTs and OTs. There are many more options. There are a group of codes which are very tempting to the pediatric therapist and in some instances may seem to be appropriate. But keep in mind that for the purpose of medical billing, you must be treating a condition that is considered to be medical in nature and that is directly related to what you treat. These codes are in the F80, F81, F82, F83 and F84 range. Check these codes out but read them carefully. Please read beyond the title. They relate to disorders that are psychological and cognitive in nature and they apply to children. Understandably, since we often work with children who have additionally been diagnosed with developmental delay, we assume that this is a disorder that we treat. Just as with a diagnosis of Down Syndrome, cognitive disorders associated with developmental delay are not disorders that we directly treat, although our treatment of other disorders can certainly affect cognitive and psychological disorders in a positive way. As an example, ICD code F82 is 'specific developmental disorder of motor function'. But if you read the clinical information it specifically states that this impairment in motor development is not due to a medical condition. It includes the conditions of 'clumsy child syndrome', 'developmental coordination disorder' and 'developmental dyspraxia'. In these conditions there is no known underlying physical cause. F82 may be a risky code to use in billing for PT or OT services. However the ICD code F80.2 is 'mixed receptive-expressive language disorder'. The clinical information section states:

- A disorder characterized by an impairment in the development of an individual's expressive and receptive language capabilities which is in contrast to his/her nonverbal intellect. The impairment may be acquired (i.e., due to a brain lesion or head trauma) or developmental (i.e., no neurological insult).

This diagnosis would seem appropriate for many of the children treated by the speech language pathologist. However, be prepared for a denial. There are other codes which are more accurately used for children with associated conditions or diagnoses. Some payers deny all F codes as 'developmental delay' and interpret it to mean the child is just behind. If this is the case, contact the payer and ask if there is an accepted code for the condition you are treating or offer an alternate code and ask if that would be accepted.

The pediatric SLP should use "R" codes for billing purposes whenever possible. These codes should be used for any child that has another known related (otherwise known as secondary) medical condition such as autism, Down syndrome, or any diagnosed medical disorder which could account for the child's need for your service.[9] You don't bill for the secondary condition, instead you bill for the condition you are treating (the primary condition), but the secondary should be present. Here are some examples:

R41.841   Cognitive communication deficit *(due to organic disturbances and intellectual disability)*
R47.01   Aphasia (not related to CVA)
R47.02   Dysphasia (not related to CVA)

---

[9] American Speech-Language-Hearing Association. (2016). *2017 Coding & billing for audiology and speech-language pathology*. : Author.

R47.89   Other speech disturbances *(this code includes speech production and processing concerns)*

R48.2   Apraxia (not related to CVA) *this code does not require a secondary condition*

R48.8   Other symbolic dysfunction *(the description refers to conditions related to aphasia)*

R62.51   Failure to thrive, failure to gain weight

R63.3   Feeding difficulties, feeding problem

R13.11   Oral stage dysphagia (food sensitivity)

I69.022   Dysarthria following non-traumatic subarachnoid hemorrhage *(since the treatable condition is included with the known medical diagnosis you don't need to use an "R" code for this condition)*

At the time of this writing, the ICD-10 codes are still new and we are learning which codes most closely meet our requirements as well as how these codes are interpreted by payers. These codes are also being refined and sometimes redefined over time. Remember, many health insurance payers have a policy against reimbursement for developmental conditions, because they define 'developmental delay' as 'the child is just behind and will catch up without therapy'. But some F80 code definitions open up the possibility that the cause of the speech impairment may be due to a medical condition. Become familiar with these codes, but I recommend that you do not use them unless the condition you are treating absolutely will not fit under a category which is more concretely described.

Regardless of the diagnosis code you decide to use, remember that the diagnosis must be a good match with the specific treatment you are providing or payment will be denied. For instance, for SLPs, the diagnosis R13.11 oral stage dysphagia is not a match for CPT Code 92507 'Treatment of speech, language, voice, communication and/or auditory processing disorder', however, it is a match for CPT Code 92526 'Treatment of swallowing dysfunction and/or oral function for feeding'. If you mismatch your codes, you will likely be denied payment and will have to take extra time to correct your claim and wait for delayed reimbursement.

CPT Codes

I cannot reproduce the CPT[10] code book for you in this chapter. Your professional organization, APTA, AOTA, and ASHA can help you access a modified CPT Code book specific to your profession. However, I will give you guidelines to know, as well as some precautions.

Let's start with Speech Language Pathology. The two main codes you would use for treatment are 92507 and 92526, defined above. These are untimed codes, meaning each code represents one complete treatment session. You generally cannot include timed codes with either of these treatment codes as each code represents an all-inclusive session. The code 97532 'cognitive training' is a timed code to be billed in 15 minute increments. SLPs can bill this code. However, it cannot be billed in conjunction with 92507 or 92526. The Rule of 8's is the rule you must use for billing timed codes. This rule is described later in this chapter.

A few years ago, you may have experienced more flexibility and differences in rules for billing with various payers. However HIPAA rules and electronic billing as well as the National Correct Coding Initiative (NCCI)[11] require that everyone plays by the same rules. So even though you may not be able to bill the way you used to, at least you will know that at this time, the rules are the same for everyone and thus less confusing.

Pediatric PT's and OT's generally use timed codes when working with children. CPT codes 97110 'Therapeutic Exercise', 97112 'Neuromuscular re-education', and 97530 'Therapeutic activities' are codes commonly used in pediatrics. You should refer to the CPT code book for specific definitions. It is expected that you will provide home exercise programming for your patient and/or caregivers during your therapy session. The training time falls under the specific treatment code(s) that describes the emphasis of your treatment. There is no separate code for parent training, patient education or home exercises. All of these codes are timed codes. Each code is billed in 15 minute increments. Because your sessions are billed in timed codes, your treatment notes must always include the time spent providing services. If you include an untimed code in your session, such as a re-evaluation or

---

[10] American Medical Association. (2016). *Coding and Payment Guide* (2017 ed.). Salt Lake City, UT: Optum360, LLC.

[11]

https://www.cms.gov/Medicare/Coding/NationalCorrectCodInitEd/index.html?redirect=/nationalcorrectcodinited/

an evaluation then your notes must include the time spent during the evaluation as well as the time spent in direct treatment. Your billed treatment time does not include patient down time such as a diaper change or a 'time out', unless it is part of the treatment.

There are rules around how to bill your timed treatment codes. This is sometimes called the Rule of 8. Below is the explanation provided by the Department of Health and Human Services 2006 and also in the CPT code book (2017)[12]:

> ### C. Counting Minutes for Timed Codes in 15 Minute Units
> *When only one service is provided in a day,* providers should not bill for services performed for less than 8 minutes. For any single *timed* CPT code *in the same day measured in 15 minute units,* providers bill a single 15-minute unit for treatment greater than or equal to 8 minutes *through and including 22* minutes. If the duration of a single modality or procedure *in a day* is greater than or equal to 23 minutes t*hrough and including 37* minutes, then 2 units should be billed. Time intervals for *1 through 8* units are as follows:
> ### Units Number of Minutes
> *1 unit:* ≥ *8 minutes through 22 minutes*
> *2 units:* ≥ *23 minutes through 37 minutes*
> 3 units*:* ≥ *38 minutes t*hrough *52* minutes
> 4 units*:* ≥ *53 minutes t*hrough *67* minutes
> 5 units*:* ≥ *68 minutes t*hrough *82* minutes
> 6 units*:* ≥ *83 minutes t*hrough *97* minutes
> 7 units*:* ≥ *98 minutes t*hrough *112* minutes
> 8 units*:* ≥ *113 minutes t*hrough *127* minutes
> The pattern remains the same for treatment times in excess of 2 hours.
> *If a service represented by a 15 minute timed code is performed in a single day for at least 15 minutes, that service shall be billed for at least one unit. If the service is performed for at least 30 minutes, that service shall be billed for at least two units, etc. It is not appropriate to count all minutes of treatment in a day toward the units for one code if other services were performed for more than 15 minutes.*
> *When more than one service represented by 15 minute timed codes is performed in a single day, the total number of minutes of service (as noted on the chart above) determines the number of units billed.*
> *If any 15 minute timed service that is performed for 7 minutes or less than 7 minutes on the same day as another 15 minute timed service that was*

---

[12] American Medical Association. (2016). *Coding and Payment Guide for the Physical Therapist* (2017 ed.). Salt Lake City, UT: Optum360, LLC.

also performed for 7 minutes or less and the total time of the two is 8 minutes or greater than 8 minutes, then bill one unit for the service performed for the most minutes . This is correct because the total time is greater than the minimum time for one unit. The same logic is applied when three or more different services are provided for 7 minutes or less than 7 minutes.

The expectation (based on the work values for these codes) is that a provider's direct patient contact time for each unit will average 15 minutes in length. If a provider has a consistent practice of billing less than 15 minutes for a unit, these situations should be highlighted for review.

If more than one *15 minute timed* CPT code is billed during a *single* calendar day, then the total number of *timed* units that can be billed is constrained by the total treatment *minutes for that day.*

Pub. 100-02, chapter 15, section 230.3B Treatment Notes indicates that the amount of time for each specific intervention/modality provided to the patient is not required to be documented in the Treatment Note. However, the total number of timed minutes must be documented. These examples indicate how to count the appropriate number of units for the total therapy minutes provided.

Example 1 -
>   *24 minutes of neuromuscular reeducation, code 97112,*
>   *23 minutes of therapeutic exercise, code 97110,*
>   *Total timed code treatment time was 47 minutes.*

See the chart above. The 47 minutes falls within the range for 3 units = 38 to 52 minutes.

Appropriate billing for 47 minutes is only 3 timed units. Each of the codes is performed for more than 15 minutes, so each shall be billed for at least 1 unit. The correct coding is 2 units of code 97112 and one unit of code 97110, assigning more *timed* units to the service that took the most time.

Example 2 -
>   *20 minutes of neuromuscular reeducation (97112)*
>   *20 minutes therapeutic exercise (97110),*
>   *40 Total timed code minutes.*

Appropriate billing for 40 minutes is 3 units. Each service was done at least 15 minutes and should be billed for at least one unit, but the total allows 3 units. Since the time for each service is the same, choose either code for 2 units and bill the other for 1 unit. Do not bill 3 units for either one of the codes.

Example 3

33 minutes of therapeutic exercise (97110),
7 minutes of manual therapy (97140),
40 Total timed minutes

Appropriate billing for 40 minutes is for 3 units. Bill 2 units of 97110 and 1 unit of 97140. Count the first 30 minutes of 97110 as two full units. Compare the remaining time for 97110 (33-30 = 3 minutes) to the time spent on 97140 (7 minutes) and bill the larger, which is 97140.

Example 4 –
18 minutes of therapeutic exercise (97110),
13 minutes of manual therapy (97140),
10 minutes of gait training (97116),
8 minutes of ultrasound (97035),
49 Total timed minutes

Appropriate billing is for 3 units. Bill the procedures you spent the most time providing. Bill 1 unit each of 97110, 97116, and 97140. You are unable to bill for the ultrasound because the total time of timed units that can be billed is constrained by the total timed code treatment minutes (i.e., you may not bill 4 units for less than 53 minutes regardless of how many services were performed). You would still document the ultrasound in the treatment notes.

Example 5 –
7 minutes of neuromuscular reeducation (97112)
7 minutes therapeutic exercise (97110)
7 minutes manual therapy (97140)
21 Total timed minutes

Appropriate billing is for one unit. The qualified professional (See definition in Pub 100-02/15, sec. 220) shall select one *appropriate CPT code* (97112, 97110, 97140) *to bill since each unit was performed for the same amount of time* and only one unit is allowed.

NOTE: The above schedule of times is intended to provide assistance in rounding time into 15-minute increments. It does not imply that any minute until the eighth should be excluded from the total count. The *total minutes of* active treatment counted *for all 15 minute timed codes* includes all direct treatment time *for the timed codes. Total treatment minutes-- including minutes spent providing services represented by untimed codes— are also documented. For documentation in the medical record of the services provided see Pub. 100-02, chapter 15, section 230.3: Documentation, Treatment Notes.*

Simply put, if your entire treatment session was provided in timed minutes then divide the time by 15. That will give you the total number of units you can bill for the session. If the remainder is 8 or more, you can add one more unit. If you use a variety of treatment codes, you must decide how to proportionately divide the codes for billing within the total treatment time. The time spent with untimed codes should not be included in your calculations. However it should be reported as time additional to the timed treatments provided. You might report the total time of the session as well as the timed portion of the session. I usually break it down and report timed-code period and untimed-code period.

BILLING 'CO-TREATMENTS'

Sometimes the patient benefits from the simultaneous treatment of two types of therapies, for instance PT and Speech, or PT and OT. Even though the time of each therapist is required for the entire session, CPT code rules do not allow billing of a full session by both therapists. You are billing for the patient's time in treatment, not the therapists' time. The Speech Therapist can bill one unit of 92507 as usual and regardless of time, however, the PT and OT, may only bill a portion of the session. So a combined one hour session with PT and OT can be billed as a half hour session by each therapist (or other agreed upon proportion). The patient cannot be billed for two hours of treatment during a one hour period. A combined one hour PT and Speech session could be billed as a half hour session by the PT and one session of Speech therapy. You can decide upon different proportions, but you must both agree and document accordingly. The CPT code book simply says "if multiple procedures are appropriately performed concurrently, they should not be billed as done consecutively".[13]

BILLING HOME EXERCISE TRAINING

As therapists, we know that home exercise (activity) training or coaching is the key to success in any therapy treatment plan. If you have ever worked with adults in an outpatient setting, you know that much of what you do with patients is to insure

---

[13] American Medical Association. (2016). *Coding and Payment Guide for the Physical Therapist* (2017 ed.). Salt Lake City, UT: Optum360, LLC. Page 10

that they are clear on what to do on their own for continued progress. You coach the patient each step of the way through every technique or exercise.

The same rule applies to working with infants and children, except instead, you must coach the parent or caretaker. We all know that what happens at home on a daily basis is what will contribute best to the success of your care. As the professional, you know what activities will work best and what techniques will be the safest and most effective for each particular patient.

There is no additional code for billing home exercise training. Instead, you are expected to bill the treatment code most closely related to the focus of the training/treatment. It is expected that your entire treatment session includes home program training. Some payers are beginning to request documentation that caregivers are complying with recommendations.

Sometimes a parent may require an exceptional amount of time for your training. This could be due to the parent's own disability or other factors. As long as the focus of your treatment plan and home exercise program is on the needs of the child, you can bill for treatment of the child. In this case, your documented treatment plan would include the extra training time or modifications that may be required for caregiver training.

Coding Modifiers and Special Circumstances

There is a system of two-digit modifiers that has been developed to allow the provider to indicate that a particular service or procedure has been provided under altered circumstances. This allows the payer to recognize that a modification in reimbursement should be considered.

The intricacies of using modifiers when billing, is beyond the scope of this manual. More detailed information on the use of modifiers can be found in the CPT code book. However, there is one modifier that you should be aware of early on. Some healthcare payers may have a policy that does not allow a re-evaluation as a payable service. This is because the re-evaluation has been misinterpreted by some therapists to mean a progress report. I went into detail on this concept in Chapter 4, Documentation. It is possible, however, to help the payer understand that your re-evaluation does, in fact, meet the standards of a true evaluation. This can be done with modifier '59'. You would use Modifier 59 with your re-evaluation code. This would designate your re-evaluation as a distinct procedural service. An audit would require that you produce a written re-evaluation that meets the standards described in Chapter 4.

There are other circumstances where you may want to use Modifier '59', depending upon services provided and the policies of the payer.

If you are interested in providing telehealth services, Modifier '95' was added in 2017 and is meant to alert the payer that there is an altered circumstance of service.

Evaluate and Treat

Occupational therapists, physical therapists and speech therapists can provide and evaluation and treatment during the same session. This has been discussed in earlier sections of this chapter. But for simple reference it will be repeated and further clarified in this section.

In the case of speech therapists, you can simply bill for one unit of your treatment code and one unit of your evaluation code, since neither are timed codes. You must have a separate evaluation document and separate treatment documentation.

In the case of physical therapy and occupational therapy you will be combining an untimed evaluation or re-evaluation code with your timed codes. Technically, reimbursement of your evaluation code is not based upon time spent with the patient during your evaluation. However, if you combine the evaluation with treatment, your time in treatment must be documented. You can document this is two ways. Your treatment note can document total time of session with a separate notation of treatment time. Or you can document time spent in evaluation and time spent in treatment. For instance, I may write "35 min eval, 25 min tx". The place to document time would be on your treatment note. I usually write up my treatment notes and include "see evaluation dated mm/dd/yy" so the reviewer will know there is a separate evaluation document.

Travel Time

If you live in the western states or rural areas, you know that travel time can be a big chunk of your day. You may be used to getting reimbursement from your school district or early intervention agency for mileage and/or time travelled. There is no means of charging medical payers for travel time. Your reimbursement is intended to include all overhead costs for providing treatment. It is up to you to limit your overhead costs, whether it is the cost of running a well-equipped facility or the cost of travel to your service location. Either situation can get out of hand.

If you are billing your services to a medical payer for a child you are seeing as a result of an early intervention referral, it is certainly an option for you to request reimbursement from the EI agency for time or distance travelled. The EI agency may have a policy regarding travel reimbursement. Sometimes there may only be reimbursement for extreme distances since the EI agency may have difficulty finding a provider otherwise.

If you are seeing a patient privately, you can always have a policy to only see patients within a certain distance of your office, limiting your expenses. You can also have a policy that, for example, there will be an additional flat rate fee for distances beyond a certain range, explaining that this fee will cover the additional time and expense required for travel.

You are allowed to charge additional fees for extended travel because this is not a service reimbursed by a medical payer. However, a policy such as this may cause a patient to receive services elsewhere. Also, if the patient has Medicaid, some state Medicaid agencies will cover the cost of patient travel to receive a medical treatment. Make sure the patient family understands that this may be an option before they pay unnecessary extra dollars for your service.

Keep in mind that mileage (not time) travelled during work is still a tax deductible expense as of this writing. However, if you are reimbursed for your mileage elsewhere, you may not additionally claim it as a tax deductible expense.

Telehealth

Make certain you are up to date on your state's requirements for telehealth. As of this writing, it is generally accepted that regardless of where you happen to be at the time, you should be licensed in the state where the patient is at the time of treatment. State licensure is designed to protect consumers, so they only have control over services provided within state lines. This could change over time, especially if our healthcare system becomes more nationalized.

Not all states have licensure regulations around telehealth. If yours does not, then the next level of authority would be your professional organization. Some payers have restrictive rules around the location of the provider (office versus other) and the location of the patient (office, clinic, home, etc) at the time of treatment. Make certain you are aware of those restrictions before providing service.

In Colorado, the state early intervention program requires that providers receive specific training in provision of telehealth services. I took the training and found it very helpful. Even though state licensure may not yet require training, you must meet the requirements of the referring agency or the payer. When in doubt, always adhere to whichever policy is strictest. You must still adhere to HIPAA standards for privacy for telehealth, so don't plan on sitting at Starbucks and providing therapy online.

When billing for telehealth, you use the same codes as you would use for your other treatments. The place of service code for telehealth is 02 and you should use that code rather than 11 (office) or 12 (patient home). To distinguish your telehealth visit from another visit, you may also be required to include a 'modifier' code in conjunction with your bill. Modifier 95 is listed in the CPT code book as the appropriate modifier for telehealth. But it is possible that a payer may have a different recommended coding strategy. So if you would like the option of providing telehealth service to a patient, call the payer to ask how you should bill for that service. There may be some creative policies out there since this is a relatively new approach to treatment. For example, at the time of this writing, Colorado Medicaid requires the addition of modifier code TG for telehealth services.

Exclusions

If you are a physical therapist you provide physical therapy. If you are an occupational therapist you provide occupational therapy. If you are a speech therapist you provide speech therapy. All of these are services that are usually paid by all healthcare payers. However, sometimes therapists provide a separate and distinct service that may be specifically listed as "exclusion". In other words this service is not covered by the payer. You may be surprised at some of the non-covered services. These may seem to be arbitrary, but you need to pay attention. You should also know that some services that may be covered in a hospital setting may not be covered in an outpatient setting. You can go to any payer website and learn if a service you would like to provide is excluded. This does not mean it isn't mentioned, instead you should see a specific statement that the treatment is not a covered service.

Not all payers are the same. Some services that are not covered by one payer are services that are clearly supported by another payer. As we receive continuing education throughout our careers, it can be difficult to parse out what part of our treatment is one technique or another. Pay attention to the focus of your treatment for billing purposes. Are you working on strength, posture, communication, balance? Surprisingly, some payers are uncomfortable with settings---as if progress could not possibly be made with treatment on a horse or in a pool. But other times, the payer focuses on specific techniques such as craniosacral therapy as "unproven" treatment.

If a service is specifically listed as uncovered, you should not bill the payer for providing that service. Any time spent providing that service should not be included in your total treatment time.

Denials and Fraud

One of the biggest concerns I hear from therapists who have never done their own billing, is that they are worried about payment denials and being accused of fraudulent billing if they make a mistake.

In my experience over the years, most payment denials occur because of mistakes on the bill. For instance, an incorrect diagnosis code or your treatment doesn't match the condition descriptor. If you use a general medical diagnosis, you may get a denial that looks as if your service is not covered for a patient with that diagnosis. Understand that the assessment of your billing is to determine/verify that the condition is specifically treatable by your service.

Also, I have found that the payer makes mistakes, some payers more than others. In one instance, I became so frustrated with making frequent phone calls to request the payer correct their own mistakes, that I quit taking new patients with that insurance.

With regard to being accused of fraud, the only time that would happen would be if it was clear that you were consistently billing for services not provided. Now, that can be interpreted many ways. For instance, if you are not a qualified physical therapist and you are billing for a physical therapy evaluation, then that is fraud. If the payer policy says they will not cover a particular service provided by an assistant and you bill for the service anyway, then that is fraud. If you consistently bill for one-on-one service when treatment is actually in a small group, then that is fraud.

Most often, if you are billing incorrectly, due to incorrect coding, you won't be accused of fraud, you will just be asked to reimburse the payer. Sometimes, you can simply correct the mistake with a corrected bill and other times, there is just no way around it and the money must be returned. Don't worry. If you follow the guidelines in this guide and the CPT code book, you will not likely bill incorrectly.

Chapter 7:
Those Dang PT and OT Evaluation Codes

I decided to add a chapter on selection of evaluation codes for PTs and OTs, simply because they seem to be a source of consternation among some therapists. It is frustrating that we have to learn a new system, but that happens sometimes. When you think that a PT who evaluates an athlete with knee pain has been getting paid the same as a PT who evaluates a patient with head trauma and multiple concerns, it begins to make sense.

The rules for the new PT and OT evaluation codes help the provider remember to focus on the problem oriented evaluation as described in Chapter 4. This is especially important for pediatric therapists who previously or recently have worked in the school setting or in the early intervention setting where evaluations and communications with families are supposed to take a strengths-based approach.

The medically based evaluation should be concise and focus on patient difficulties that we hope to improve with therapy. In addition, we must document concerns that we may not treat but that may affect our treatment approach or interfere with our treatment.

The new PT and OT evaluation codes requirements are slightly different from each other, so pay attention to your discipline-specific documentation requirements.

One approach to assigning a code to your evaluation is to write up the evaluation and then start counting the elements of the evaluation that meet the specific code requirements. Start with the requirements for the high complexity code (97163 or 97167) and if your evaluation and patient do not and cannot meet those requirements, look to the moderate complexity code. If your documentation cannot meet all of the requirements of the moderate complexity code, look to the low complexity code requirements. Keep in mind that at the very least, your evaluation must meet the requirements of the low complexity evaluation. You must make sure you are truly writing a problem focused evaluation and including all of the basic required elements.

Reimbursement will be different for your evaluation based upon the complexity assigned, so you must be prepared for the payer to review your evaluation to verify the complexity.

Assignment of complexity to the code is not just dependent upon the depth and extent of your evaluation. The documented complexity and status of the patient is also an important part of this assignment. The complexity of the patient is usually included in the introductory history and background of the patient. Many of the children we work with are highly complex, but we must remember to document the specific concerns that influence our treatment.

REQUIRED ELEMENTS OF THE PHYSICAL THERAPY EVALUATION

Physical therapy evaluation CPT codes 97161, 97162, 97163 and re-evaluation 97164

Patient background and history

This section of the evaluation is basically the introduction of the patient. Be as brief as possible while, at the same time, including all relevant information. It may be helpful to create a checklist for yourself to remember to address information that may affect the outcome of your service. I have created a chart which you can see in Appendix I "Physical Therapy Evaluation Codes" at the back of this book. I have also added a downloadable PDF to my website at www.smallpatientpractice.com. You can use that chart as a guide or create one of your own. Just remember, as you are writing your evaluation, do not include information that is irrelevant to your service provision. Here are some things that might be included in your introduction:

- Patient age and birth history, including prematurity, oxygen needs at birth, known traumas

- Reason for referral to your service
- Known medical diagnoses such as Down Syndrome, cerebral palsy, cerebral hemorrhage, GERD, seizure disorders
- Current durable medical equipment such as a walker or wheelchair, orthotics
- Other therapy services or health professionals patient sees
- Known medications
- Complicating factors such as heart or respiratory disorders, impending surgeries, vision or hearing impairments
- Medical disorders that may affect the rate of progress such as heart conditions, JRA or cancer treatment
- Known mental or cognitive disorder
- Other symptoms that may affect progress such as skin rash, chronic allergies, healing fractures, general health
- Patient social support such as living with family, foster care or institution

In order for the physical therapist to consider assigning the high complexity code (97163) the evaluation must include a history of the current concern with "3 or more personal factors and/or comorbidities"[14] such as the ones listed above, that affect your care plan.

Objective Examination/Assessment

This section of the evaluation is your opportunity to document your objective observations and testing results.

The physical therapist is expected to document standardized tests and measures results that demonstrate problems with "body structures and functions, activity limitations, and/or participation restrictions."[13] A high complexity exam requires 4 or more tests evaluating any of these areas. These tests and measures may include, for example, assessment of gross symmetry, ROM deficits, strength deficits, patient size compared to peers, balance, gait and locomotion patterns, transitions, coordination, motor control, or motor learning. Your training allows you to determine whether these skills are normal or abnormal. Cardiovascular and

---

[14] American Medical Association. (2016). *Coding and Payment Guide for the Physical Therapist* (2017 ed.). Salt Lake City, UT: Optum360, LLC. Page 83.

pulmonary problems, swelling, and skin integrity should also be reported. The pediatric therapist should also note whether communication and interaction with people and objects is age appropriate.

Don't let the word 'standardized' lead you to believe a standardized developmental evaluation is required. In fact, it is not. However, keep in mind that each skill element within a comprehensive developmental test has been standardized to specific ages. So you can report on elements that are specific to your needs for the PT evaluation. For instance, the Hawaii Early Learning Profile[15] expects a child to achieve cruising between 9.5 and 13 months. You can report that the 15 month old child is not yet able to move holding on to furniture as would be typical for a child his age. If the skills are at age level but the quality is a concern, you can test speed, safety, distance, motor patterns, etc. Just as there are standardized procedures for measuring strength and ROM, there are many standardized procedures for testing mobility such as the "Timed Up and Go", "Timed Floor to Stand", "Dynamic Gait Index", "50-foot Walk Test" and "30-second Walk Test".[16] You can also report on gait patterns, stride length and width, postural control during gait. You do not necessarily have to compare the test results to same age peers. Instead you can use the testing criteria and get a baseline for your evaluation and measure progress or set goals using the data. There are many other useful tests including tests for balance (Pediatric Balance Scale) and tests for trunk control (Segmental Assessment of Trunk Control).[17]

Patient presentation

In addition to the elements you include as part of your evaluation, the status of the patient is a vitally important aspect to determining whether your evaluation is of high complexity.

In order for the physical therapist to assign a high complexity value to the evaluation, the patient must have a "clinical presentation with unstable and

---

[15] Revised Hawaii Early Learning Profiles [Measurement instrument]. (1085-2004). Retrieved from www.vort.com

[16] Resource: top 10 walking tests for school-based PTs. (2017). Retrieved July 31, 2017, from www.seekfreaks.com

[17] Resource: top 9 functional balance tests for school-based PTs. (2017). Retrieved July 31, 2017, from www.seekfreaks.com

unpredictable characteristics".[18] This is as far as the definition goes at the time of this writing. There are some characteristics that we frequently see in the outpatient pediatric caseload that could make the clinical presentation unstable and unpredictable:

- Heart conditions which affect patient performance
- Hydrocephalus not yet or recently shunted
- Seizure disorders
- Certain behavioral disorders
- Respiratory disorders
- Severe digestive or swallowing disorders including GERD
- A cluster of symptoms and concerns that have not yet been given a diagnosis
- Progressive disorders such as ALS or muscular dystrophy at certain stages
- Acute inflammation in JRA
- Recent or upcoming symptoms that will impact function
- Post-surgical instabilities

Any of these concerns, and others, has the capacity to wreak havoc upon a physical therapy care plan and should be seriously considered as you determine whether the patient's condition is stable. This does not mean the presence of one of these conditions renders the patient's condition necessarily unstable. The condition could simply be a comorbid concern. What you must consider is whether the condition is under control and predictable at the time of your evaluation.

Clinical Decision Making

The high complexity physical therapy evaluation requires "high complexity clinical decision making using standardized patient assessment instrument and/or measurable assessment of functional outcome".[17]   So basically, the evaluation measurements you used in your evaluation should have helped you assess the patient's deficits and needs, create a care plan and establish goals which can be meaningfully measured to determine progress. A complex patient requires a higher level of clinical decision making.

A shortcut reference tool for assigning a complexity code to your evaluation is available in the APPENDIX I. You may also download, print and share a PDF copy of this document at www.smallpatientpractice.com.

---

[18] American Medical Association. (2016). *Coding and Payment Guide for the Physical Therapist* (2017 ed.). Salt Lake City, UT: Optum360, LLC. Page 83.

The Physical Therapy Re-evaluation (CPT code 97164)

The re-evaluation is more extensive than the standard re-assessment of patient status that occurs at every visit. This formal document will include a review and update of the patient's history, including how much physical therapy has already been received and response to treatment, including progress toward or barriers impacting goal attainment. Tests and measurements must be included, as well as a revised care plan and updated goals resulting from the tests and measures if appropriate.

REQUIRED ELEMENTS OF THE OCCUPATIONAL THERAPY EVALUATION

Occupational therapy evaluation CPT codes 97165, 97166, 97167 and re-evaluation 97168

As with the physical therapy description of evaluation earlier in this chapter, the following will focus on the high complexity evaluation and the reader can refer to Appendix J "Occupational Therapy Evaluation Codes" to determine how to meet the requirements of the moderate or low complexity evaluation.

Patient background and history

The coding description for this section of the evaluation is referred to as the "occupational profile including medical and therapy history".[19] The term "occupational profile" refers to the patient's reason for referral to OT, with a brief overview of contexts and environments that support and hinder activity.

In order for the occupational therapist to consider assigning the high complexity code (97167) the evaluation must include a "review of medical and/or therapy records and an extensive additional review of physical, cognitive or psychosocial history related to current functional performance".[6] The word 'extensive' is not defined, so it is up to the judgement of the therapist and the payer to determine what this means. It stands to reason that a patient with a more complicated history would require a more extensive background review. This does not mean you are required to provide lengthy documentation, but it does mean that your documentation should reflect that an extensive review was performed. A list of topics

---

[19] American Medical Association. (2016). *Coding and Payment Guide for the Physical Therapist* (2017 ed.). Salt Lake City, UT: Optum360, LLC. Page 85

you might consider is included in the physical therapy evaluation section of this chapter. You can also look at Appendix J.

Objective examination/assessment

The CPT coding description refers to this segment of the evaluation as assessments that identify performance deficits relating to physical, cognitive or psychosocial skills. The 'high complexity' code requires at least 5 performance deficits relating to those skills and resulting in activity limitations or participation restrictions.[20] This should be pretty straight forward for the pediatric OT when looking at motor and self-help skills using individual skill elements standardized to age level. Keep in mind that each skill within a standardized developmental test has been tested and compared to same age peers. Some test protocols such as the chart included in the Revised Hawaii Early Learning Profile[21] provide expected age ranges for individual skills achievement.

The number of deficits is the number of occupations or performance skills that are being impacted and will be addressed in the plan of care. The AOTA recommends that these skills may include ADL activities such as sleep, play, social participation and subcategories such as bathing, toileting, dressing and eating.[22] Each of these ADL categories and others can be counted as a performance deficit.[23]

Sensory concerns should be reported as comorbidities even if these concerns are the primary reason for the child's performance deficits. However, remember to be specific in your identification of concerns and avoid using the word "sensory" in your evaluation because many insurance payers do not understand the word and may deny

---

[20] American Medical Association. (2016). *Coding and Payment Guide for the Physical Therapist* (2017 ed.). Salt Lake City, UT: Optum360, LLC.

[21] *Revised Hawaii Early Learning Profile* [Measurement instrument]. (1985-2004). Retrieved from www.vort.com

[22] American Occupational Therapy Association. (2014). OT practice framework - table 1 (occupations). Retrieved from http://ajot.aota.org

[23] Brennan, C., & Glennon, T. J. (2017). Frequently asked questions (FAQs) for correctly choosing new evaluation codes for pediatric OTs. Retrieved from https://www.aota.org/Advocacy-Policy/Federal-Reg-Affairs/Coding/new-OT-CPT-evaluation-cods.aspx

payment for your entire service if it looks like you are going to provide a service that is not covered. Be concise regarding your concerns and how the behaviors may interfere with progress. For instance, you can report that the child is hyper-responsive to light touch and tends to handle the stress by withdrawing. You should then describe how this comorbidity affects the child's performance deficit or deficits (such as dressing and/or play). This is a comorbidity that can affect progress toward goals and may require treatment modification.

Comorbidities should be part of the evaluation process if in the therapist's judgement they affect occupational performance.[24]

Patient presentation

In order for the occupational therapist to assign a high complexity value to the evaluation, the patient must have comorbidities that affect performance. Comorbidities could include, but are not limited to behavioral concerns, specific sensory deficits, communication concerns, vision, health or physical impairments. Additionally the patient must require significant assistance (physical or verbal) or modification of tasks in order to complete an evaluation component. In the world of pediatrics this means the patient would require assistance or modification in order to achieve an age appropriate task.

Clinical Decision Making

The high complexity occupational therapy evaluation (97167) must be of high analytical complexity, which includes an analysis of the patient profile, analysis of data from comprehensive assessment(s) and consideration of multiple treatment options. Many, if not most pediatric occupational therapy evaluations, meet this standard. But remember, all of the elements described in each segment of the occupational therapy evaluation in this chapter must be met and documented in order to designate 97167 as the evaluation code.

---

[24] Brennan, C., & Glennon, T. J. (2017). Frequently asked questions (FAQs) for correctly choosing new evaluation codes for pediatric OTs. Page 3. Retrieved from https://www.aota.org/Advocacy-Policy/Federal-Reg-Affairs/Coding/new-OT-CPT-evaluation-cods.aspx.

Appendix J may be a helpful shortcut tool with required elements of information for each designated OT evaluation code. You may also download, print and share a PDF of this chart from www.smallpatientpractice.com.

The Occupational Therapy Re-evaluation (CPT code 97168)

The re-evaluation is not the standard assessment of patient status that occurs during every visit. Instead, it is a formal document that reviews and updates the patient history and changes to medical and social status. It may include new tests, especially if functional status has changed. You should also include progress toward or barriers to goal attainment. The re-evaluation usually includes updated goals and may include a changed plan of care.

The Small Patient Practice

Chapter 8:

Reading the Explanation of Benefits (EOB)

When you are paid for your medical services, the payment will be accompanied by an Explanation of Benefits, otherwise known as the EOB. Read this statement carefully or you may miss some important information.

Each payer has its own EOB format. Sometimes it would seem you need extra intuitive powers to understand what it is saying. Most often the EOB is straight forward.

An EOB with No Payment

If the EOB arrives without a check for payment of your services, you must pay special attention. The EOB will usually list the Date of Service and the Amount Billed. If nothing was paid one of a few things will be listed. For instance, it could say that the amount allowed was $100.00, but that $100.00 was applied to the deductible and so you must bill the patient for the full amount.

More Information Needed

When no payment is made, and if the total allowed is not applied to the deductible, you must carefully read the EOB to determine what is needed. Payment may be denied because of incorrect billing or coding. If you can't figure out the problem, call and ask. On the other hand, the EOB could state that payment is pending receipt of medical records including physician referral, treatment notes and plan of care (your evaluation). In this case, you simply photocopy those documents and send them with a copy of the EOB requesting the documents and put them in the mail. Make sure you document when those documents were mailed, in order to keep track of your reimbursement trail. Sometimes reimbursement could be pending additional information requested from the patient. In this case you must wait for the patient to provide the requested information to the payer. Patient families don't always read the fine print on their insurance statements, so you may have to do some coordinating to make sure everything gets done. I would call the insurance company to determine the status of that request if you have not received a another response within 30 days.

Amount Allowed

The Amount Allowed is usually not the same as the amount billed, but sometimes it is. Don't simply trust that the 'Amount Allowed' is correct. First make sure that all of the codes you billed have been counted. Then, if everything is accounted for, you can usually trust that the payer has correctly determined what they (the payer) determines to be allowed reimbursement. If you have a contract with the payer and are a network provider, you must accept the Amount Allowed as payment in full. If you do not have a contract with the payer, then it is your option to accept the Amount Allowed as payment in full. Or you can decide to accept nothing less than the amount you billed as payment in full.

Amount Allowed vs. Amount Paid

The Amount Allowed is not the same as the Amount Paid. If the patient is required to pay a copayment or coinsurance then the Amount Paid is the amount paid by the healthcare payer and the patient will be required to pay the balance. The total of the amount paid by the patient and the healthcare payer should be the amount allowed. If the patient has a fixed copayment for each visit, you may collect the copayment at the beginning of each session and so the amount paid by the healthcare payer would be the balance of the Amount Allowed.

Amount Paid vs Amount Billed

If you bill more than the payer allows, you may not ultimately be paid the full amount billed. There are some contingencies. You are required to bill the patient the difference between the amount paid and the amount allowed. If you have a network contract with the payer, you cannot bill the patient an amount that would reimburse you any amount over the amount allowed. That is called balance billing and virtually all network contracts forbid it.

If you do not have a network contract with the payer, then you can bill the patient the difference between the total reimbursed and the amount billed.

If you bill less than the typical amount allowed the statement will show the amount billed as the amount allowed, unless your contract says you will accept a proportion of the amount billed as payment in full.

Coinsurance vs Copayment

Some healthcare insurance payers have different verbiage for patient cost shares; here is what they mean.

Coinsurance typically means the patient plan requires that the patient pay a percent of the amount allowed or the amount billed, whichever is less. The percentage amount is fixed, but the dollar amount may be different for each visit, depending upon what services are billed.

The patient copayment is usually a fixed amount for every visit, regardless of services provided or amount billed, unless the amount billed is less than the copayment.

In the case of the copayment, since the amount is fixed, you can and should collect the copayment at the beginning of each visit. However, as a solo practitioner, I understand that this is sometimes uncomfortable and you would rather send a bill. You can ask the family which they would prefer and so if they request payment at each visit, then have a receipt available for them.

One Common Mistake

Keep in mind people who work for healthcare insurance companies make mistakes too. The codes you bill are outpatient therapy codes. Even though the amount reimbursed for your service code does not change, there is a box for 'location of service' on the bill. When you list '12' patient home as the location, sometimes the person processing your claim will simply look at the 12 and not the specifics of your treatment codes. This means your treatment session could be processed as a home healthcare visit rather than an outpatient therapy visit. It may be tempting to ignore this, but if it appears that your reimbursement was for a home healthcare visit, you may want to clarify this. Here are some possible issues that could arise from the misclassification of your visit:

1. Since you are not a home healthcare agency, a medical review of your records could determine that you are not meeting documentation and service requirements of a home healthcare agency.
2. Reimbursement allowable amounts are usually different for home healthcare and you may be overpaid. A payment audit could determine that you must reimburse amounts overpaid.
3. There may be different policies for the number of outpatient visits allowed, versus the number of home healthcare visits allowed and this could result in an incorrect allowance of services.
4. The payer may deny your services as not allowed because your service does not meet the requirements for allowed home healthcare services.

If it appears that your service may have been misclassified, just call and ask for clarification. If the rules for your services and the reimbursement and patient cost share amounts are consistent with expected outpatient therapy service costs, then everything should be fine. However, if the EOB statement is contrary to what is expected, you should pursue this.

For instance, if your service was denied due to lack of authorization and you already know that the patient is allowed outpatient services without an authorization, you can be pretty certain that your service was misclassified. The person who processed your claim may not realize that outpatient services can be provided in the home. In this case, you should specifically cite the Medicare policy which states that outpatient services in the home are allowed. I have provided a copy of a letter I once sent to a payer for successful reclassification of my services in Appendix K. If you are billing on the payer's website, there may be a means for you to request a review through online communication. You should always cite the related Medicare rule. Just understand that not all payers are required to comply with Medicare policy. However, once a payer knows something is allowed by Medicare, they usually accept the policy.

Another glitch you may run into regarding misclassification of your services is computerized processing of your bill. In most cases this is not a concern and the payment systems automatically process your claim as an outpatient service whether provided in an office or the patient's home. However, the occasional payer has the system set up so that all services provided in the home (listed as number 12 on the claim form), will be classified as home health services. In this case you will not be paid correctly, if at all. When this has happened to me, I have called the payer, explained what service was provided and asked what I should do to get paid. Once the claims processor understood that this is a legitimate service, I was told to always put the number 11 (office) on the claim regardless of the actual location. When I asked to have this in writing, my request was denied of course, but I documented our conversation and kept the information on file so that I would have some justification for why I needed to bill the payer in this way.

Special billing circumstances for specific payers will happen on occasion. Once you learn what they want, payment usually goes smoothly. When I work with a new payer, I try to submit my first bill as soon as possible just so I can make sure there will be no special issues. If there are, I must figure out what to do to adapt. Even if payment goes smoothly, it can suddenly change due to a policy or payment system change. This is just part of the thrill of self-employment.

IN SUMMARY

Basically, the EOB is the statement from the healthcare payer. This statement describes the responsibilities of all of the parties. The patient is required to pay the amount designated. The provider (you) is required to submit requested paperwork. Finally, the EOB states the amount the healthcare payer is required to pay. You should verify that everything that is stated is what you expected and that it is correct.

Once you have marked your visit as paid and received the patient share of the reimbursement, then you can file the EOB in the patient file. Never discard the EOB. If you get an audit, you will want this information at hand.

Chapter 9:

Billing the Patient

Most healthcare insurance plans require that the patient share in the cost of services provided. This means that you are required to bill the patient for his or her share of the costs. There is no getting around this. You must bill the patient. There are Federal laws as well as state laws in place to enforce this rule. See Appendix L.

If the patient has a supplemental insurance, Medicaid or other insurance coverage, then you can bill that entity instead. When you bill these medical payers, you bill them the same way you bill the primary insurance payer, with the CMS 1500, either electronically or with a paper bill. In this case, when you bill, you must report the amount already paid. This is Box #29 of the CMS 1500. If billing electronically, you would list the amount paid in the area designated in the electronic format.

Balance Billing

There are often at least two totals to consider when billing the patient. The total 'amount billed' is the amount you charged and billed the patient for your services. The 'amount allowed' is the amount the payer (insurance company) recognizes as the maximum amount allowed for your service. If you indicated that you will 'accept assignment' in Box#27 on form CMS 1500, then you have indicated that you will accept the 'amount allowed' as payment in full for your service. In this case you bill the patient the difference between the 'amount allowed' and the amount paid by the insurance company.

If you have a contract with the payer, then your contract likely stated that you must accept the 'amount allowed' as payment in full. In this case you are not allowed to bill the patient any more than the payer 'allowed' for your service on that date. If you bill up to the full 'amount billed' rather than the 'amount allowed', this is called 'balance billing'. Balance billing is not allowed when you have a network contract.

If you do not have a network contract with the payer, then you can bill up to the full amount of your charge for services. You can accept what the insurance company pays and you can bill the patient the difference. Be certain the patient family understands they are responsible for the full amount of your charge.

Sometimes the patient will ask you to accept what the payer allows, even though you do not have a contract. It is your prerogative to accept that request.

Consistent Billing

Regardless of the payer, the amount billed per code should be the same amount billed for every payer. The payers will pay what they allow, but they expect you to bill fairly and consistently.

Cash Based Practice

You do have the option of running a cash based practice. This means you would charge the patient a flat rate for your service and it would be up to the patient to file the paperwork for reimbursement from their insurance company. You would still need to create a bill with the appropriate codes so the patient can seek reimbursement. Another option would be to collect full payment from the patient for your services and then bill the insurance company. Leave Box 13 blank and healthcare insurance payment will be made to the patient.

The main drawback to running a cash based service is that most clients will prefer to go elsewhere. There are plenty of providers who are willing to make service delivery as simple as possible for families.

One advantage to running a cash based service is that you can charge lower fees, since you will not have the additional cost and payment delay associated with healthcare insurance billing.

How to Bill the Patient for Copayments and Deductibles

When I bill the patient, I like to make the bill as simple to understand as possible. If you have received bills for medical services, choose one to use as a model. I have an example of a simple bill format in Appendix M.

It is easiest to keep track of your bills and payments if you bill on a schedule. Also, if your patient does not reimburse you immediately, he should receive another bill within 30 days of the last one. If a second bill is sent, be certain to indicate that this is the second bill.

When you are billing the patient as a solo provider, it is rare that a patient would not pay his share of costs. You can remind the patient that you are required to bill the copays and the patient is required to pay them. If the patient has fallen behind, you can offer a payment plan to help him manage the costs spread over time.

Reducing Patient Cost

There are a few ways you can reduce patient costs. One way would be to reduce your fees. In most cases, if the insurance company pays less, then the patient pays less. This is not the case if the patient must pay a fixed amount per visit.

You are allowed to set a policy for financial need, which would allow certain families to pay you a fraction of their required co-pay. You must have a policy in place and the patient must give you something in writing that you can keep on file. You can establish an annual income with relation to the poverty threshold or median income for your community. You can also accept a letter explaining extenuating circumstances which make payment difficult for the patient's family for a period of time. Most importantly, you cannot extend this cost break to everyone. This policy should only cover special circumstances.

Patient Refusal to Pay

It is rare that a patient's family will refuse to pay. If you send a bill and thirty days later send another billed labeled 'SECOND BILL', this is likely the most you will have to do for payment. If after the second thirty days you get no response, you should call and speak directly to the responsible party. Ask if there is a reason she has not yet paid the bill or if she has any questions about the bill. Sometimes an explanation may be provided by the patient allowing you to offer either a discount or a payment plan.

If at any time you are concerned that the patient is not going to pay his share of the treatment cost, it is your option to discontinue services with a recommendation for other providers who can continue treatments. You must recommend another provider, because you do not want to be accused of abandoning the patient. You can also put the service on hold until the bill is paid. In either case, there is no guarantee that you will be paid. It is your option to contract with a collection agency. The reputable collection agency will accept payment in the form of a percentage collected. You can also write it off.

Generally, if you stay on top of your billing, pick a consistent time of month when you will take care of patient billing, you will be paid. If it looks like you don't keep track of billing, by sending late or sporadic bills, you are setting yourself up for delinquent payments.

This is your livelihood. Run your practice in a professional manner and you will be rewarded with a consistent and reliable income.

Chapter 10:

Wording Your Medical Records

A lot of what we do as therapists is misunderstood by non-therapists. In pediatric rehabilitation, what looks like play is really a combination of strengthening, coordination, endurance, balance and/or any other concern you are addressing. How you communicate this in writing is important and can mean the difference between payment and non-payment.

School based therapists are required to word their documents in a way that is understood by teachers, parents and any other interested parties. Services provided under Early Intervention are expected to be worded in terms of family concerns and priorities. For both School and Early Intervention services, the reports must focus on the child's strengths and 'next steps'.

The medical evaluation and report must be problem-focused and must use medical terminology that is accepted and understood by other medical providers. Your evaluation must convince the reader that your treatment is medical in nature and medically necessary. Medically necessary means that if the service is not provided, the patient's medical condition could decline. A patient's medical condition can decline if, for example, he cannot walk, if he cannot feed himself, if he cannot tell you something hurts. You work with a 'patient' and you must get to the point with the problem(s) you will be addressing as a therapist. Your professional education has prepared you for this.

There are Early Intervention agencies around the country now requesting that you bill healthcare payers for medically necessary services provided under the Early

Intervention program. In some cases this will mean you must provide two separate evaluations. The first evaluation may be the developmental assessment required to qualify the child for services under Early Intervention. The second evaluation will be your discipline specific, problem-focused medical evaluation. If the Early Intervention agency is doing the medical billing, the therapist will need to provide the medical evaluation separate from the family-friendly IFSP. Most health insurance payers will not or cannot change their payment policies to cover services which are not medically necessary.

The following are some hot topics regarding medical documentation.

Developmental Delay

As I mentioned in an earlier chapter, many insurance companies have a policy that does not cover 'developmental delay'. They interpret developmental delay to mean the child is simply 'behind' and will catch up given enough time.

'Developmental delay' is not a diagnosis. It is a symptom that when used alone, explains nothing. It is up to the professional therapist to determine if there is an underlying and treatable medical condition. The therapist must focus on the medical condition(s) when writing the evaluation. The only acknowledgment of development should be in terms of 'expected level of function' which is impaired as a result of the medical condition.

When you evaluate the child from your professional perspective, you must determine if there is an underlying condition which may be contributing to the delay and which is treatable by your profession. Furthermore, you must document this condition in a medical and problem-focused way. Here are some examples of medical conditions which can interfere with a child's function:

1. Jeremy lacks sufficient strength and muscle control to support himself on his arms for activities such as crawling and getting up to sitting.
2. Cassidy has mild right sided weakness which will interfere with the attainment of gross motor skills such as crawling and walking.
3. Aiden has impaired protective reactions and this contributes to his fear of falling, interfering with mobility skills.
4. Susie has difficulty with the organization and coordination required for self help skills.
5. Matthew is unable to follow single step directions or make simple requests known.

6. Tess has good receptive communication, but lacks sufficient oral muscle coordination and strength for word formation.

Note that each of these examples is worded in a way that clearly spells out the problem(s) that can be addressed by your profession. They are worded in a way that another medical professional would acknowledge as a disorder which can be corrected by your medical service.

Sensory Integration

Sensory Integration therapy has been defined, redefined, maligned and misunderstood as a treatment approach. Many payers have a policy that does not cover Sensory Integration as 'it is unproven' as a treatment approach. This is due to at least one study that was reported several years ago. I have seen the term 'sensory integration' used in many ways, most incorrectly. The provider of sensory integration requires specific training in this approach to treatment.

Even if your treatment is focusing on other areas of concern, if you even use the words 'sensory' or 'sensory integration', your entire treatment plan could be denied as not allowable by some payers.

If you have a patient that has a sensory concern in one or two areas, it is best to specifically describe the condition if you plan to treat it. Most so called 'sensory' issues are really common disorders addressed by professional therapists, including vestibular dysfunction, poor coordination, abnormal sensation, and gravitational insecurity (poor balance and protective reactions). If the medical reviewer understands what you are specifically treating, your treatment may be approved.

If you will not be treating a sensory condition, there is no reason to document it, unless you believe it may affect the patient's progress. In this case, you should be specific and say, for instance, 'Johnny's agitation with light touch and fear of falling may slow his progress in the attainment of gross motor skills'. Avoid jargon which is only understood by therapists.

Progressive Disorders

The treatment of children with progressive disorders can be confusing. In spite of the progression of the disease, the child can learn and gain skills as the rest of his body is functioning as it should. Children with progressive disorders grow, develop, play and socialize.

The therapist must help the child develop strategies which will compensate for losses which occur as a result of the progression of the disorder. These compensations will change as the child develops and the disease progresses. Additionally the therapist must teach the family protocols for and monitor protection of joint integrity, safety, use of assistive technology and equipment.

Your documentation should be specific and goal oriented. You should never use the passive words 'maintain' or 'prevent'. Maintenance and prevention do not usually warrant your specialized care. Your goals should be realistic and functional for that child. Your evaluation should focus on current functions and the issues you plan to address.

Remember, you are not treating the progressive disorder. You can't. You are treating the conditions which arise as a result of the disorder and the conditions should be the focus of your documentation.

I once participated in a panel presentation sponsored by the American Physical Therapy Association in New Orleans. The topic was 'Physical Therapy Management of Children with Progressive Neuromuscular Disorders Across the Lifespan'. My role in the presentation was to offer medical billing and documentation suggestions. As I sat through the presentation, I was inspired to write a plan of care for each case study presented, using wording that would most effectively explain what the therapist wanted to accomplish. Here are some examples:

1. A seven year old with Duchenne Muscular Dystrophy, need to train the family in a home exercise program that includes stretching to 'maintain' the child's ability to walk.
   Suggested Plan of Care: Physical Therapy to delay the progression of contractures and preserve adequate muscle strength to move and function independently, with patient and family follow through on recommended activities.

2. A nine year old boy with Duchenne Muscular Dystrophy with frequent falling secondary to muscle weakness and joint tightness. Would like to continue walking a little longer.
   Suggested Plan of Care: Physical Therapy home exercise program to help the patient preserve sufficient muscle strength and joint range for

walking at least one more year. Help the patient and family with the transition to wheelchair mobility.

3. A seventeen year old with Duchenne Muscular Dystrophy, s/p spinal fusion, is concerned that he is losing current skills.
   Suggested Plan of Care: Physical Therapy for training in a pulmonary program, home exercise program for joint integrity, and recommended activities to support health and well-being. Work with the technology required for independent mobility and function at work and in the community.

4. A one year old with Spinal Muscular atrophy. The therapist wants to maintain skin elasticity and joint range of motion, promote increased circulation, provide sensory input and decrease pain.
   Suggested Plan of Care: Physical Therapy to teach compensatory strategies and alternative movement to improve function. Provide home exercise program to provide contracture control, skin integrity, healthy circulation and pain control.

5. A 15 month old with Spinal Muscular Atrophy having difficulty sitting while playing.
   Suggested Plan of Care: Physical Therapy to provide strategies and adaptations for functional dynamic and static sitting with family follow through on recommended care.

The above examples were given during my presentation in New Orleans. A Speech Therapy example for a child with a progressive disorder such as Werdnig-Hoffman's Disease would be as follows: **Speech/Language Therapy to provide training and strategies for use of a communication device to help patient communicate basic needs.**

Notice that none of these plans includes the passive sound of 'maintenance' and 'prevention'. There is nothing passive going on in these plans. The provider is clearly addressing the medical and functional needs of the child at that period of time in the child's development and with the progression of the disorder. As a medical provider, you must clearly communicate the active and essential elements of the service you provide.

I don't typically include my goals in my 'Plan of Care' summary paragraph. I list them separately and earlier in the evaluation. My 'Plan of Care' summary paragraph typically includes my planned treatment frequency and duration with 'parent follow-through on recommended activities'. The above examples were simply for economy of time during the presentation. Your documentation style is not important, as long as all of the required elements are present and clearly understood.

IN SUMMARY

* Use medically oriented words that describe the condition you are treating.

* Don't get sidetracked describing conditions that have little relevance to the service you are providing.

* Don't use 'catch-all' terms that may flag your treatment plan as non-covered.

* Your plan of care should be proactive and realistic.

Chapter 11:

Troubleshooting

Patient Needs Adaptive Equipment

Every payer has different rules regarding the purchase of adaptive equipment. I find it best to work with the vendor. Hopefully your community or a community nearby has a medical supply vendor who can order equipment. You should use a vendor in-network with your patient's payer, if at all possible. The vendor typically takes the measurements, gets the approval of the payer and places the order. The vendor will want your input regarding the most appropriate equipment required for the patient and the patient's environment. Sometimes I am very particular about the equipment or device I want my patient to have and I will speak to or meet with the vendor to make sure this happens.

The purchase of durable medical equipment will require a physician prescription. This is often procured by the vendor, but sometimes I will fax a specific request to the physician and ask that a prescription for that device be faxed to the vendor. I will even include a photo of the device and justification. Either you or the family can request that the prescription be faxed to the vendor of choice. I will sometimes give the physician a heads up that a patient may require a certain piece of adaptive equipment, including orthotics. This way the physician knows I am on board with the request. Sometimes a patient will go to a specialty clinic and a physician will order equipment before I am even considering it and in most cases that is fine. In the end, the therapist will be the one helping the patient use the device, so if I believe the equipment will not work in the patient's environment, I will take steps to have the order modified.

If requested, it will be your responsibility to provide a written justification for the equipment. The justification must be from the patient perspective. When equipment is ordered for the patient, the equipment must meet the patient's needs. It is not for the convenience or the safety of the caregiver. You should recommend equipment that will help the patient access the community, provide safety to the patient, or promote the health or increase the level of independence of the patient. It may help to provide examples of how the equipment will be used. It may also help to explain why that particular piece of equipment, or one like it, will best meet the patient's needs. It is appropriate to include features of the patient's environment or the specific community the patient must access (for instance hills and rugged terrain).

Patient's Healthcare Policy has a Restricted Number of Visits per Year for Service

Some healthcare policies include a fixed number of visits for your service per year. For instance, the payer may allow 50 Physical Therapy visits per year, or as little as 20 each of outpatient PT, OT and Speech. Some healthcare policies allow a fixed number of combined visits. For instance, the payer may allow a maximum of 60 outpatient PT, OT and Speech combined visits per year. If this is the case, it is essential that you find out if the patient is receiving or has received any other services during that year. In this case you will need to coordinate your services with other providers and the patient (family) may have to decide which service should be cut back or discontinued.

Policies are sometimes flexible, allowing additional services, if a medical review of your records supports the need. However do not count on this as there are policies which make no allowances. You can call the payer and ask if they make allowances for special circumstances that require more therapy, for instance, an unexpected surgery.

Health Insurance Payer Denies Payment

There are multiple reasons why your services may be denied payment. If you receive a denial, do not assume that the denial is correct or based on policy. For instance, if you bill electronically and get a denial, look closely at the reason for denial. Let me give you some examples of possible reasons for denials and simple solutions.

1. **Services denied due to lack of authorization**
   If you contacted the healthcare payer before beginning services and were told that your outpatient therapy services do not require prior authorization, there is a good chance your services were misclassified as home healthcare services. See Chapter 8 regarding solutions to this problem.

2. **Services not covered for developmental delay**
   If you simply submitted a bill for your services, there would be no way for the payer to know if you are treating the child simply because of developmental delay. Some payers may have an automatic response set up for children under a certain age. It is up to you to call and tell the payer that you are not seeing the child for developmental delay, rather for a medical condition. When you call, the payer will either request documentation (a copy of your evaluation) for review of medical necessity, or may simply pay you.

3. **Services not covered for educational needs**
   As in the previous example, if you simply submitted a bill, the payer cannot really know if the child you are treating has a medical condition. Speech Therapy is often questioned for medical necessity and this may be an automatic response for patients below a certain age. It is up to you to call and tell the payer you are seeing the child for a medical condition. At this time, a copy of your evaluation may be requested.

4. **Payment denied due to 'diagnosis not a coverable condition'**
   This can happen if you mistakenly appointed the wrong diagnosis to the service provided. For instance, if you are a Speech Therapist and you listed 'dysphagia' with your speech therapy treatment code. In this case, you simply need to submit a corrected claim. Details of how to do this are in Chapter 5.

5. **Payment denied or delayed pending receipt of documentation**
   If you were not specifically asked to submit documentation, the payer could be waiting for other types of documentation from the physician or the patient. You may need to call about this one.

6. **Payment denied or delayed pending additional information from recipient**

The recipient is the patient. Sometimes the payer is asking the patient if he has other forms of insurance coverage, or other health information. You may want to contact the patient (family) and make certain he has complied with the request.

Reimbursement is Delayed

States exercise varying levels of jurisdiction over the practices of health insurance companies within their state. Many states require reimbursement, or a response to billing within a certain time frame, for instance, 30 days. When you submit a bill, whether electronically, or by mail, you should note what day the bill was submitted or mailed. Payment should be received within 30 days or whatever time limit is required by your state. Contact your state professional association for specific information. Here are some reasons why payment is delayed and what you should do about it.

1. Payment was sent to the family.

   This may happen if you forgot to indicate on the bill that the patient authorized payment directly to you. I once experienced working with a payer that routinely pays the patient for your services if you are a non-network provider. This can create problems both for you and the patient. If the payment was made to the patient, you will receive nothing from the payer. When you call the payer, you will be told payment was made to the patient. Ask the payer how much was paid and the date of the payment. You will then call the patient (family) and request a copy of the statement and the full amount of the payment be sent to you. The alternative would be to bill the patient for the date(s) of service.

2. Additional documentation required

   This was discussed in Chapter 8 and on the previous page.

3. Payment delayed pending review of medical records

   If your medical records were requested, the payer may request additional time for review of your records.

The Healthcare Payer Wants Reimbursement

Don't panic. Many healthcare insurance companies take steps to ensure your service meets their requirements for medical necessity prior to payment. Some situations can occur which will require partial reimbursement of amounts previously paid. It is possible that your state has a policy prohibiting a payer to request reimbursement for their own mistakes after a certain period of time. Your state professional association may be able to help you with this. Here are some situations which may occur:

1. Your services were overpaid as network services rather than non-network services.

    In this case, once you reimburse the healthcare payer, you can bill the patient for the corrected copayment amount which is the responsibility of the patient.

2. Your services were incorrectly paid as home healthcare services rather than outpatient therapy.

    In this case, once you reimburse the insurance company the amount overpaid, the patient may have a new required payment. Depending upon the corrected allowable payment, you may additionally need to reimburse the patient a certain amount. Either way, you would need to submit a new statement to the patient with an explanation.

3. A medical audit reveals you billed incorrectly

    You should be able to submit a corrected claim and this may result in a 'break even' claim with no additional money exchanged. The corrected claim could also result in a required partial payback or additional income.

Policy Denies Payment Because Child Getting Services in School

This occurs most frequently with federally related payers rather than private insurance companies. No payer wants to pay for services which are already provided elsewhere. Many people may not realize that school based services are intended to meet the educational needs of the child, but do not typically fulfill the medical requirements of service provision. School systems do not have to acknowledge a doctor prescription for therapy services which are not educationally related. The need for school based therapy services can only be determined by the student's Individualized Education Plan (IEP).

The payer may want to see the IEP to determine if school based services are meeting the patient's medical requirements for service provision. In most cases a review will reveal the services are insufficient to meet the patient's medical needs. It doesn't hurt to additionally get a statement from the school Special Education Director to reiterate that the school district is not responsible for meeting the child's medical needs. Parents are usually willing to help you with this.

Payer Policy Does Not Cover Reported Service

Once you have exhausted all other possible mistakes or clarifications, it is possible that the healthcare payer has a policy prohibiting your particular service for the condition you are addressing.

It is possible that the sharing of additional outside evaluations will support the need for your service. For instance, a hearing test could reveal a hearing loss or an MRI could reveal an intracranial hemorrhage.

If you are certain you have all necessary and appropriately documented medical information and believe that the healthcare payer's policies are flawed, the patient (family) can submit an appeal. Each payer will have guidelines for submitting an appeal. This is often a lengthy process and really should be the last possible option. Make sure the family pays attention to timelines required for the appeal.

You can help the patient by submitting supportive research and documentation (consensus statements, practice guidelines, journal articles, etc).

Look for local patient or parent advocacy groups to assist the family with the appeal process. Condition-specific organizations (such as the Muscular Dystrophy Association) may have useful information. The family should also request that the physician provide support in advocating for the service.

I recommend that therapy services be discontinued while you are waiting for the appeals process. The family needs to be motivated to pursue the appeal.

Payer Reimbursement is Insufficient

It is possible that the allowed reimbursement amount from a particular payer is insufficient to cover your costs. In fact, you may believe that if all of your payers reimbursed this amount, you would change careers. I get it. I have seen it.

Since you are self employed, you get to decide which healthcare payers you will accept and which you will not. You may not discriminate against patients based upon their race, color, religion, sex, or national origin however you can refuse to accept patients who carry a healthcare insurance with which you do not want to work.

You are running a business and it is imperative that your business survives in order for you to continue practicing.

You may have a policy that you will not accept patients who are covered by a particular insurance company or payer. If you are already seeing a patient that has the insurance you have decided to no longer accept, you can do one of a few things. You can explain to the patient (family) that you can no longer accept his insurance, but will help him find another provider. You can explain that you will no longer accept his insurance, but offer to accept cash payments and your patient can seek reimbursement from his insurance. You can also decide that you will no longer accept new patients with that particular insurance, but will continue with the patients that you currently are seeing.

Another option is to restrict the number of patients who are covered by a particular payer. For instance, if you are a Medicaid provider and want to continue seeing Medicaid patients, but are concerned about the reimbursement amount, you can create a policy that your patient caseload will only include up to a certain percent of Medicaid patients. This will allow you to keep your business alive and still see a certain number of Medicaid patients. The rest of your practice will be supported by patients whose payers will keep your income in balance. Not all state Medicaid programs reimburse insufficient amounts, this was just an example.

SUMMARY

If I have a problem with reimbursement, I find it most helpful to begin with a phone call and see what I can learn.

When a mistake is made in billing, it can always be corrected.

When I think I've seen it all and am prepared for anything, something new will happen. New policies and rules turn up all of the time. Sometimes the policies apply to your service and sometimes they don't.

CHAPTER 12:

Your Office, Your Practice and HIPAA

The following is a series of suggestions for running your office and your practice. I have learned some things by trial and error and learned other strategies from fellow solo practitioners.

It is easiest to keep your medical records, communications and scheduling in order if you have a dedicated office. If your office is in your home, remember you must keep patient records private and you must have locking file cabinets. The technology devices you use with patient information must be password protected. There can be tax advantages to having a dedicated office in your home so speak to your tax advisor. There can be tax advantages to having a dedicated office in your home. Speak to your tax advisor.

Healthcare payers require a listed office location, even if you provide services in the patient's home. A post office box cannot be listed. Keeping this in mind, your home office address may be revealed on any network provider lists.

Since HIPAA rules and technology have become major players in running a health related service, this chapter will begin with that topic and then move on to other aspects of running your office.

Health Information Privacy

Since the first publication of this book, there are a few updates and requirements from the Department of Health and Human Services. HIPAA stands for Health Insurance Portability and Accountability Act of 1996. Everything you want to know about HIPAA can be found on www.hhs.gov/hipaa. This law was first established in the wake of electronic technology that allowed transmittal of patient health information (PHI). As technology changes, it is updated as needed. The website will help you determine what aspects of the rule apply to your practice or particular setting and it is a good idea to intermittently check on updates.

Even if you are an employee and not a practice owner, if you do any portion of your work on your home computer, including documentation of patient contact, telehealth, billing or email, you should insure you meet the requirements for privacy.

The HIPAA website has a new set of publications called the Security Series. It is a reader friendly series of HIPAA security documents known as the Security Rule Educational Paper Series and includes seven downloadable documents for providers.

1. Security 101 for Covered Entities
2. Administrative safeguards
3. Physical safeguards
4. Technical safeguards
5. Organizational, Policies and Procedures and Documentation Requirements
6. Basics of Risk Analysis and Risk Management
7. Security Standards: Implementation for the Small Provider

Here are some highlights of the things the small practice owner should understand regarding HIPAA:

- The privacy rule applies to all PHI whether electronic, written or oral.
  - Most of us are familiar with the policy of obtaining written permission from families before communicating with other healthcare providers or entities. We also understand that we must be careful not to be overheard by others when speaking of PHI. There are however, new rules regarding electronic protections.
- The security rule refers to electronic forms of PHI, including transmission or storage

- One of the most frequent vulnerabilities is loss or theft of an unprotected laptop or cell phone. If you have PHI on your device it must be password protected and have a shut-down feature.
- A healthcare provider must have administrative, technical and physical safeguards to protect the privacy of PHI from intentional or unintentional disclosure
- The healthcare provider's own risk analysis, security analysis and financial analysis should support safeguards which are implemented.
    - Clearly, safeguards will look different for a large multidisciplinary clinic versus a solo provider, even though the standards are the same for both.
- You must have a Business Associate Agreement (BAA) or contract with your billing entity (clearinghouse) verifying that you will both be HIPAA compliant.
    - I found one on my agency's website, ready for me to sign. The billing agency I currently use is www.officeally.com because there is no charge for non-Medicare patients. You may occasionally need to update the agreement as the provider requires.
- Any documentation of policies or agreements must be available for HIPAA review for up to 6 years.
    - So even if you update your agreement, keep the old for your files.
- You must make every effort to protect PHI from loss whether due to natural causes or theft (and let's not forget computer crashes), so you must have a means of backing up all PHI.
    - The most reliable means of protecting electronically stored PHI from loss is through an online backup system or 'cloud'.
- Now you must have a formal Business Associate Agreement (BAA) with your online backup provider if you keep any PHI on your computer or mobile device. You can still use an external backup device instead. Just make sure you update it regularly.
    - As of this writing, the iCloud is not HIPAA compliant and will not sign a BAA. This means that you must disconnect the iCloud from your device if you keep PHI on it, even if you have a separate external device. It is worth shopping around for a HIPAA compliant online backup company. There are some good ones at a

fair price. I currently pay $5 a month for mine. Just don't forget to download and sign the BAA.

- Your email is another risk to PHI so if you MUST use it to transmit PHI, then you must put a few things in place. Once again, you should have a signed BAA with your email provider. You should also get patient consent to transmit information by email. The consent should include an explanation of the risks associated with transmitting PHI through email.
    - HIPAA compliant email services are a growing industry. Most require a low monthly fee, but I did find a free one, called Medtunnel which I have not tried, but which may meet your needs.
    - I don't email PHI, but I do use online fax. Some fax companies transmit through your email. It seems as if your email should be HIPAA compliant if you use this method, but I haven't seen any rules for that. Apparently if the online fax company you use is HIPAA compliant and especially if it provides a BAA, the encryption and precautions of the online fax company take care of needed protections. As of this writing I have found three online fax companies which will sign a BAA: srfax.com, faxage.com, and sfax.com. You may be able to use your secure online backup provider as a means of transmitting PHI safely as well, so check out your options.

Although it sounds complicated to become HIPAA compliant, once you have your own policies, plans and permission forms in place, you don't really have to think about it anymore. It is a good idea to review everything once a year, just to make sure you didn't miss anything and to make sure you are compliant with your own policies.

FAX

Most insurance companies and doctor offices communicate by fax. It is convenient to be able to receive physician referrals by fax. You can also fax copies of your evaluations and any other requested documents to physicians and payers. You have a few options here. You can have a fax machine with a dedicated phone line. You can also have a fax machine that is hooked up to your office phone, which only works when you turn it on. I have switched to using online fax. I listed three HIPAA compliant online fax companies which will sign a BAA in the previous section. Shop around. With online fax I have been given a fax number which receives faxes 24 hours a day. The faxes are sent to my secure email address and I can open and print them whenever I choose. To send out faxes using this system, your printer must have a scanning option available. The best thing about using online fax is it requires no additional equipment.

Phone

If you have a family, you should not use your home phone as an office phone. If a physician office, insurance company or patient calls, they must be able to leave messages or speak directly to you. You always want to present a professional image with your telephone response and voicemail. If you do not want to pay for an additional office phone line, you can use a cell phone. Just make sure the settings are professional and that the caller doesn't have to listen to a trendy or musical message. Always answer your phone in a professional manner.

Scheduling

You must be self-disciplined to run your own practice. When you schedule patients, remember to allow for driving time, if you see patients in their homes. Travel time is not reimbursable and you should not include it as part of your treatment time. You should set up blocks of time for your patient scheduling so that you can have blocks of time set aside for medical documentation, billing and necessary communications in your office. The best way to stay on top of paperwork is to document all of your treatment sessions before the end of the day. Some therapists document their treatment sessions in the last minute or two of each visit. Write up all evaluations on the day of your first visit.

Set aside one or two periods of time per month for billing. You should bill families for copayments and deductibles at or near the same time of month every month. This will allow you to more easily keep track of payments and late payments.

Most therapists I know who run full time practices from their homes set aside at least a half day a week to take care of special communications, authorization requests, phone calls, billing and any unexpected requests.

The drawback to running an office from your home is that if you do not give yourself a work schedule, you will begin to believe you work all of the time. Set up your work day and office hours and abide by them as closely as possible. If you are working 12 hours a day, you may be seeing too many patients, or you may need to schedule more efficiently.

The beauty of running your own business is that you can schedule important personal activities into your work week. For instance, you can schedule an hour at the gym into your workday.

Reliability

Besides being a good therapist who works well with patients and families, you must be reliable. Families must be able to count on you to be there regularly. If you must be late, call ahead. If you have a schedule conflict, try to offer a makeup appointment if possible. You want families to be respectful of your time and you should be respectful of their time.

No Shows

The nice thing about bringing your therapy to the family home is that cancellations are less frequent. We do work with high risk children and they do get sick frequently, so cancellations are not completely avoidable. You can establish a written policy that requires families to give you at least 24 hours advanced notice for cancellations or they will be asked to pay a fee (a fixed amount). Beware of a policy such as this, however, as you could be inviting more cancellations. The family may be afraid that they might have to cancel, so they cancel anyway.

I always thought I might eventually have a policy requiring payment for no shows or late cancellations, but so far the problems have been minimal, so I haven't had to set anything up.

A 'no show' is when you arrive at the house for your scheduled visit and the patient is not there or is sick, or the patient does not arrive at your office for his scheduled appointment. This is rare and in most cases, when it has happened to me, there has been a really good reason.

Parent Not Present for Appointment

One of the drawbacks to seeing a patient in the family home is there is sometimes confusion about your relationship with the family. You are a medical professional providing a medical service and all of the rules apply. The parent or guardian must be present for the treatment. If the parent wants another adult to accompany the child for the treatment, there must be signed agreements ahead of time.

Never allow the parent to leave you alone with the child while she runs to pick up a sibling from school. If the parent is going to return quickly, I offer to wait in my car (catch up with phone calls) until the parent returns, but she must bring all of her children with her. If I arrive at the house and a babysitter is there (whether adult or minor) I will not stay, unless permissions (for adult only) have been signed and arrangements have been made ahead of time. There are just too many liability issues to consider risking my license.

I have provided an example of a document that I request parents to sign when they want another adult to accompany their child in their absence. See Appendix N. I have also provided an example of a Memorandum of Understanding to be signed by the accompanying adult in Appendix O. The accompanying adult must understand my expectations with regard to their presence during my sessions. As therapists we all understand the necessity and value of follow through on recommended activities and exercises. We need an adult to accept responsibility for this.

Coordinating Services With Early Intervention Agencies

If you have the opportunity to provide services as a result of a referral from an Early Intervention Agency, I recommend it. Your local Early Intervention Agency is a great referral source and you will have the opportunity to expand your network of professional contacts. Depending upon your relationship with the Early Intervention Agency, you can bill healthcare insurance as a solo practitioner, you can contract with the EI Agency for direct reimbursement, or you may even be employed by the Early Intervention Agency. I have done all three at one time or another.

If you are a licensed PT, OT or SLP in your state, it is of vital importance that you provide services within the dictates of your license, first and foremost. There is never a situation where your work environment overrides your licensure requirements for service provision and supervision. You must help referral agencies, agencies with which you contract and even supervisors understand that you can only provide services as allowed by your license. If you do not have licensure in your state, then you must provide services under the guidelines of your professional organization.

Sometimes an Early Intervention Agency will learn of a service provision approach successfully implemented in another state and will try to implement that approach in your state. What these program leaders often do not understand is that each state has its own licensure rules around service provision, evaluation protocols, supervision of non-licensed personnel, as well as service arenas. Make certain you clearly understand your own state license rules and that you abide by them; then educate others.

Paying Yourself

When you see private patients, remember that a portion of your income must go to taxes. Health Insurance Companies and other payers will send you a Tax Form 1099 at the end of the tax year and this income will be reported to the IRS. Your business expenses will help defray the amount owed on taxes so you must keep good records of your costs, including receipts. Mileage can be documented on your calendar or on a separate mileage document.

When you are just getting started, a good rule of thumb for covering your expenses and taxes is to pay yourself half of whatever you bring in and to set aside the rest in a separate account. If you are just seeing a few private patients, you do not necessarily need to open a separate checking account. You could simply open a separate savings account within your personal checking account.

If you additionally work elsewhere as an employee with a salary, you can have additional funds withheld from your employee payroll to cover anticipated taxes incurred as a result of seeing private patients. If your private practice is your only source of income, and you see several patients, you should arrange to file a quarterly tax return. A tax accountant can help you get started.

Here are some typical business and practice expenses which you should document:

Liability insurance
License fees
Continuing Education and related expenses
Reference materials
Professional dues
Costs related to professional meetings and networking
Retirement Fund
Professional Equipment and supplies
Computer
Photocopier
Fax machine and faxing costs
Phone/cell phone and costs
Office supplies
Costs related to advertising (website, business cards, etc)
Mileage
Office and/or clinic space rental or purchase
Health Insurance Premiums (may be allowed)
Disability Insurance
Taxes

Each tax year will have different rules around claiming some of these costs, but you should always be prepared. Just because these costs may be allowed as business expenses does not mean you should spend the money. If you keep your expenses down, your income will increase.

SUMMARY

Your professional reputation relies upon your integrity, reliability, and professionalism as well as your skill as a therapist.

Make certain you are up to date with regard to your state license requirements. Work cooperatively with others, but do not compromise your professional responsibility.

A well run office will support your professional success.

ACKNOWLEDGMENTS

My heartfelt thanks go to the many therapists and readers who have emailed me to request clarification and additional information on the topics provided in the first edition of this book. It has become a community project and I am happy to share information brought to my attention over the years.

I appreciate the suggestions of my dear friend Sheree York PT, DPT, PCS of Birmingham, Alabama. I also appreciate the detailed reviews provided by Sandra Slizewski Meagher PhD, OTR of Colorado Springs. Her grammatical expertise and natural curiosity are much appreciated. I am thankful for the feedback on the new CPT evaluation code charts for PT and OT received from Durga Shah PT, DPT, PCS of Atlanta, Georgia and Ellie Haddad OTR, Lori Ganz OTR, Adrienne Maxey OTR, and Kristen Merrell PT all of Colorado Springs. The work of Donna Maloney PT and Sharon Jamison SLP, CCC was vitally important to the editing of the first edition of this book and their work is still appreciated.

Finally, I appreciate the opportunities provided to me by the Academy of Pediatric Physical Therapy. I have been challenged to continue to develop myself professionally throughout my career due to my interaction with members and my participation in this excellent organization.

APPENDICES

Many of the following appendices may be downloaded from

www.smallpatientpractice.com

User: small

Password: practice

Intake Insurance Information:

Insurance Company:

Patient Name:

Date of Birth:

Parents Names:

Phone Number:

Address:

Health Insurance Sponsor Name (usually the parent whose name is on the plan):

    Is address different from above?

Insurance Benefits Phone Number:

Policy Number:

Policy Holder or Group ID:

Date: _____

Patient Insurance Plan Data

Patient name:

Date of birth:

Patient's insurance:

Co-payments:

Annual Deductible:

Network versus non-network

Insurance year:

Type of therapy: Outpatient   PT   OT   Speech

Are there a restricted number of visits per year?

       Combined with any other service?

Is Prior Auth. Needed?

Restrictions:

COMMENTS

The Small Patient Practice

Health Insurance Billing Consent Form

Health Insurance: _____

Benefits Phone number: _____

Patient's name _____Member ID_____

Patient's birth date_____ Pt Phone:_____

Patient's address_____

Physician:_____Phone:_____

Sponsor's name_____ Sponsor's date of birth_____

Sponsor's address_____

Sponsor's Phone_____Employer_____

Insured's policy group number _____Member ID_____

Other insurance_____

I consent to necessary examination procedures and/or treatment for my child by "THERAPIST NAME". I authorize the release of any medical or other information necessary to process claims. I also request payment of benefits to YOUR BUSINESS NAME HERE for services provided and claimed.

Parent signature_____Date:_____

I have been given a copy of YOUR BUSINESS NAME HERE Notice of Privacy Practices, will review it and keep it on file.

Signature_____

Your Name OR Practice Name
Business Address
Phone

NOTICE OF PRIVACY PRACTICES

Effective date

This Notice of Privacy Practices is provided to you as a requirement of the Health Insurance Portability and Accountability Act (HIPAA). It describes how I may use or disclose your child's protected health information, with whom that information may be shared, and the safeguards I have in place to protect it. This notice also describes your rights to access and or refuse the release of specific information outside of this system except when the release is required or authorized by law or regulation.

Acknowledgement of Receipt of this Notice

You will be asked to provide a signed acknowledgment of receipt of this notice. The intent is to make you aware of the possible uses and disclosures of your child's protected health information and your privacy rights. The delivery of your child's health care services will in no way be conditioned upon your signed acknowledgment.

Who Will Follow this Notice

This notice applies to all therapy services provided by YOUR BUSINESS. It also applies to office personnel and billing personnel.

Our Responsibility Regarding Protected Health Information

Your child's 'protected health information' is individually identifiable health information. This includes demographics such as age, address, email address, and relates to your child's past, present, or future physical or mental health or condition and related health care services. We are required by law to do the following:

- Make sure that your child's protected health information is kept private
- Give you this notice of our legal duties and privacy practices related to the use and disclosures of your child's protected health information,
- Follow the terms of the notice currently in effect.
- Communicate any changes in the notice to you.

We reserve the right to change this notice. Its effective date is at the top of the first page and at the bottom of the last page. We reserve the right to make the revised or changed notice effective for health information we already have about your child as well as any information received in the future. You may obtain a Notice of Privacy Practices by calling the phone number at the top of this notice.

Our System

YOUR NAME works with several agencies and referral sources. Your child's health information will be shared in the following manner:

1. Treatment—I will use and disclose your child's protected health information to provide, coordinate, or manage your child's health care and any related services. This includes disclosure to your physician or other health care providers who becomes involved in your child's care.
2. Within my office for administrative activities, quality assessment, oversight and peer review.
3. With my billing personnel and as necessary to obtain payment for your health care services.
4. With your insurance company or other payers as required for payment.
5. With the referring agency and case manager, if applicable.
6. With any other provider, school or agency with your written request.

You may request written or verbal information sharing in writing. Your request should include a specified period of time for information sharing.

Required by Law

I may use or disclose your child's protected health information if law or regulation requires the use or disclosure.

I will notify the appropriate government authority if I believe a patient has been the victim of abuse, neglect, or domestic violence.

Health Oversight

I may disclose protected health information to a health oversight agency for activities authorized by law, such as audits, investigations, and inspections. These health oversight agencies might include government agencies that oversee the health care system, government benefit programs, other government regulatory programs, and civil rights laws.

Legal Proceedings

I may disclose protected health information during any judicial or administrative proceeding, in response to a court order or administrative tribunal (if such a disclosure is expressly authorized), and in certain conditions in response to a subpoena, discovery request, or other lawful process.

Parental Access

I may disclose your child's protected information to parents, guardians and persons acting in similar legal status.

Uses and Disclosures of Protected Health Information Requiring Your Permission

In some circumstances, you have the opportunity to agree or object to the use or disclosure of all or part of your child's protected health information.

Since this service is provided in your home or other natural environments, those present during the session, including friends, family, or day care providers may hear health information regarding your child. Please notify your therapist if you do not want your child's protected health information to be discussed.

Your Rights Regarding Your Child's Health Information

You may exercise the following rights by submitting a written request to the COMPANY NAME office.

1. You may inspect and obtain a copy of your child's protected health information that is kept as a part of medical and billing records.

2. You may ask me not to use or disclose any part of your child's health information for treatment, payment, or health care operations. Your request must be made in writing. This request will be honored if we mutually agree that the restriction will not harm your child.

3. You may request that I communicate with you using alternative means or at an alternative location. I will not ask you the reason for your request. I will accommodate reasonable requests, when possible.

4. If you believe that the information I have about your child is incorrect or incomplete, you may request an amendment to your child's protected health information as long as I am responsible for and maintain this information. While I will accept requests for amendment, I am not required to agree to the amendment.

5. You may request that I provide you with an accounting of the disclosures I have made of your child's protected health information. This right applies to disclosures made for purposes other than treatment, payment, or health care operations as described in this Notice of Privacy Practices. This disclosure must have been made after 9/18/17, and no more than six years from the date of request. This right excludes disclosures made to you or authorized by you, to family members or friends involved in your child's care, or for notification. The right to receive this information is subject to additional exceptions, restrictions, and limitations as described earlier in this notice.

Federal Privacy Laws

This Notice of Privacy Practices is provided to you as a requirement of the Health Insurance Portability and Accountability Act (HIPAA). There are several other privacy laws that also apply including the Freedom of Information Act and the Privacy Act. These laws have been taken into consideration in developing policies and this notice of how I will use and disclose your child's protected information.

Complaints

If you believe these privacy rights have been violated, you may file a written complaint with the Department of Health and Human Services. No retaliation will occur against you for filing a complaint.

This notice is effective in its entirety as of DATE.

PHYSICAL THERAPY EVALUATION
Patient Name: Date:
DOB: **Primary Medical Diagnosis:**
                                                             Treatment Disorder:

Background:

Observations and Testing:

       Strength, Motor Control and Endurance

       Joint mobility/stability

       Skills:

Summary of concerns and potential for improvement:

Patient/Caregiver desired Goals/Long Term Goals:

Short Term Objectives/Therapist directed
      Date Initiated | **Objective**

Plan of Treatment

Criteria for discharge: When goals have been met and as agreed upon by family and physician.

Therapist Signature

The Small Patient Practice

Appendix F

Sample format for treatment notes

PHYSICAL THERAPY   Patient Name

TREATMENT NOTES   DOB

See goals dated	Service date	Service date
Relevant information	Activity/observations	Activity/observations
Goal		
Goal		
Goal		
Goal		
Home Program		
Narrative		
Length of Session		
Treatments	97001--- 97002--- 97110--- 97112--- Other_____---	97001--- 97002--- 97110--- 97112--- Other_____---
Initial		

Plan:_____

_____

_____

_____/_____

SIGNATURE   initial

Physical Therapy Treatment Notes and Progress

Child's Name:
DOB:
Treatment Disorder:

Date	Service Minutes	Session Treatment Notes	

Goals:
1. First goal   MET
2. Second goal   EMERGING
3. Third goal

Summary of Intervention & Progress:

Home Program/Follow-up activities for family and caregiver participation:

_____

Therapist's Signature   Date

HEALTH INSURANCE CLAIM FORM

APPROVED BY NATIONAL UNIFORM CLAIM COMMITTEE (NUCC) 02/12

| | PICA | | | | | | | | | PICA | |

1. MEDICARE ☐ (Medicare#)   MEDICAID ☐ (Medicaid#)   TRICARE ☐ (ID#/DoD#)   CHAMPVA ☐ (Member ID#)   GROUP HEALTH PLAN ☐ (ID#)   FECA BLK LUNG ☐ (ID#)   OTHER ☐ (ID#)

1a. INSURED'S I.D. NUMBER (For Program in Item 1)

2. PATIENT'S NAME (Last Name, First Name, Middle Initial)

3. PATIENT'S BIRTH DATE MM | DD | YY   SEX M ☐ F ☐

4. INSURED'S NAME (Last Name, First Name, Middle Initial)

5. PATIENT'S ADDRESS (No., Street)

6. PATIENT RELATIONSHIP TO INSURED   Self ☐ Spouse ☐ Child ☐ Other ☐

7. INSURED'S ADDRESS (No., Street)

CITY   STATE

8. RESERVED FOR NUCC USE

CITY   STATE

ZIP CODE   TELEPHONE (Include Area Code) ( )

ZIP CODE   TELEPHONE (Include Area Code) ( )

9. OTHER INSURED'S NAME (Last Name, First Name, Middle Initial)

10. IS PATIENT'S CONDITION RELATED TO:

11. INSURED'S POLICY GROUP OR FECA NUMBER

a. OTHER INSURED'S POLICY OR GROUP NUMBER

a. EMPLOYMENT? (Current or Previous) YES ☐ NO ☐

a. INSURED'S DATE OF BIRTH MM | DD | YY   SEX M ☐ F ☐

b. RESERVED FOR NUCC USE

b. AUTO ACCIDENT? PLACE (State) YES ☐ NO ☐

b. OTHER CLAIM ID (Designated by NUCC)

c. RESERVED FOR NUCC USE

c. OTHER ACCIDENT? YES ☐ NO ☐

c. INSURANCE PLAN NAME OR PROGRAM NAME

d. INSURANCE PLAN NAME OR PROGRAM NAME

10d. CLAIM CODES (Designated by NUCC)

d. IS THERE ANOTHER HEALTH BENEFIT PLAN? YES ☐ NO ☐ If yes, complete items 9, 9a, and 9d.

READ BACK OF FORM BEFORE COMPLETING & SIGNING THIS FORM.
12. PATIENT'S OR AUTHORIZED PERSON'S SIGNATURE. I authorize the release of any medical or other information necessary to process this claim. I also request payment of government benefits either to myself or to the party who accepts assignment below.

SIGNED _____ DATE _____

13. INSURED'S OR AUTHORIZED PERSON'S SIGNATURE. I authorize payment of medical benefits to the undersigned physician or supplier for services described below.

SIGNED _____

14. DATE OF CURRENT ILLNESS, INJURY, or PREGNANCY (LMP) MM | DD | YY   QUAL

15. OTHER DATE QUAL MM | DD | YY

16. DATES PATIENT UNABLE TO WORK IN CURRENT OCCUPATION MM | DD | YY   FROM   TO   MM | DD | YY

17. NAME OF REFERRING PROVIDER OR OTHER SOURCE   17a.   17b. NPI

18. HOSPITALIZATION DATES RELATED TO CURRENT SERVICES MM | DD | YY   FROM   TO   MM | DD | YY

19. ADDITIONAL CLAIM INFORMATION (Designated by NUCC)

20. OUTSIDE LAB? YES ☐ NO ☐ $ CHARGES

21. DIAGNOSIS OR NATURE OF ILLNESS OR INJURY Relate A-L to service line below (24E)   ICD Ind. |

A. |____   B. |____   C. |____   D. |____
E. |____   F. |____   G. |____   H. |____
I. |____   J. |____   K. |____   L. |____

22. RESUBMISSION CODE   ORIGINAL REF. NO.

23. PRIOR AUTHORIZATION NUMBER

24. A. DATE(S) OF SERVICE						B. PLACE OF SERVICE	C. EMG	D. PROCEDURES, SERVICES, OR SUPPLIES (Explain Unusual Circumstances) CPT/HCPCS	MODIFIER	E. DIAGNOSIS POINTER	F. $ CHARGES	G. DAYS OR UNITS	H. EPSDT Family Plan	I. ID. QUAL	J. RENDERING PROVIDER ID. #
From MM	DD	YY	To MM	DD	YY										
1														NPI	
2														NPI	
3														NPI	
4														NPI	
5														NPI	
6														NPI	

25. FEDERAL TAX I.D. NUMBER   SSN ☐ EIN ☐

26. PATIENT'S ACCOUNT NO.

27. ACCEPT ASSIGNMENT? (For govt. claims, see back) YES ☐ NO ☐

28. TOTAL CHARGE $

29. AMOUNT PAID $

30. Rsvd for NUCC Use

31. SIGNATURE OF PHYSICIAN OR SUPPLIER INCLUDING DEGREES OR CREDENTIALS (I certify that the statements on the reverse apply to this bill and are made a part thereof.)

SIGNED _____ DATE _____

32. SERVICE FACILITY LOCATION INFORMATION
a.   b.

33. BILLING PROVIDER INFO & PH # ( )
a.   b.

NUCC Instruction Manual available at: www.nucc.org   **PLEASE PRINT OR TYPE**   APPROVED OMB-0938-1197 FORM 1500 (02-12)

Physical Therapy Evaluation Codes---selection criteria and elements to consider--Pediatrics

Physical Therapy Evaluation Codes

	97161	97162	97163	97164
Include in evaluation ↓	**Low complexity evaluation**	**Moderate complexity evaluation**	**High complexity evaluation**	**Re-evaluation**
History	Relevant personal factors or comorbidities not required	1-2 relevant personal factors or comorbidities	3 or more relevant personal factors or comorbidities	Include review
Objective measures	1 -2 elements examined	3 or more elements examined	4 or more elements examined	Include examiations
Patient status	Clinically stable	Evolving clinical presentation	Unstable clinical presentation	Should report
Clinical decision making with a care plan	Low complexity	Moderate complexity	High complexity	Include revised care plan and goals as needed

If all criteria are not met within a selected CPT code, choose the next lower level.

Information on above evaluation criteria is from Coding and Payment Guide 2017 for the Physical Therapist, APTA, Optum360, LLC

Examples of What to Include in the Pediatric Physical Therapy Evaluation

HISTORY	Objective Measures	PATIENT STATUS
Age, reason for referral **Birth history:** prematurity, oxygen at birth, traumas, health of baby or mother at time of birth, drug exposures **Known medical diagnoses** including, heart, respiratory disorders, digestive disorders, neurological disorders **Current medical equipment or devices** **Current medical support** including other therapies, physicians, nursing **Known medications** **Symptoms that may affect progress,** such as	**Body systems examinations may include** (but not limited to) **Body structure abnormalities** ROM deficits, Structural deformities, posture, effect of system concerns such as pulmonary, cardiovascular, skin integrity, etc on movement and function **Abnormal motor patterns** Mobility, Transitions Postural control, Strength deficits **Specific age appropriate skills or activities not yet attained** (may use data obtained from other tests)	**Disorders such as the ones below may affect the stability of the patient and treatment course:** Heart conditions which affect patient performance Hydrocephalus not yet or recently shunted Seizure disorders not yet controlled Certain behavioral disorders Respiratory disorders Severe digestive or swallowing disorders including GERD A cluster of symptoms and concerns that have not yet

environmental awareness, skin rash, chronic allergies, healing fracture, general health **Social conditions** including home and family **Vision or hearing disorder**	**Interaction with people and objects** (indicators of alertness)	been given a diagnosis Progressive disorders such as ALS or MD at certain stages Acute inflammation such as in JRA Post-surgical instabilities

This chart Courtesy of <u>The Small Patient Practice, 2nd Ed, 2017</u>

A one page PDF download of this document is available on smallpatientpractice.com

User: small

Password: practice

	97165	97166	97167	
PROFILE AND HISTORY	Low	Moderate	High	**Examples of what to consider for the Pediatric OT evaluation**
Occupational profile, brief history, medical and therapy information related to current concern_	X			"Occupational profile" refers to the patient's reason for referral, with brief overview of contexts and environments that support and hinder activity. Consider including:
Occupational profile, medical and therapy info and review of physical, cognitive, or psychosocial <u>history related to current concern</u>		X		• Patient age and birth history, including prematurity, oxygen needs at birth, known traumas • Known medical diagnoses • Current medical equipment and devices • Known medications • Complicating factors such as heart or respiratory disorders, impending surgeries, vision or hearing impairments • Known mental or cognitive disorder
Occupational profile, medical and therapy info and extensive review of physical, cognitive, or psychosocial history related to current concern			X	• Other symptoms that may affect progress such as skin rash, chronic allergies, healing fractures, general health • Patient social support such as living with family, foster care or institution
OCCUPATIONAL PERFORMANCE ASSESSMENT				
Assessment resulting in 1-3 deficits	X			Physical, cognitive or psychosocial skills resulting in activity limitations and/or participation restrictions You may identify specific skill category deficits identified during a recent standardized developmental test, or you may test the patient for specific deficits. You may also
Assessment identifying 3-5 deficits		X		include deficits of concern reported by the patient or family. These skills are compatible with those identified with the OT Practice Framework Table 1 (available on the AOTA website) and recommended as a source for deficits in this category. Consider including: Specific play skill deficits including participation and
Assessment identifying 5 or more deficits			X	exploration Skill deficits in the areas of toileting, bathing, dressing, feeding, sleeping
COMORBIDITIES affecting performance	none	maybe	present	Comorbidities must affect patient performance and should be part of the evaluation process. They may include but are not limited to: Behavior, specific sensory concerns, communication, vision, hearing, health, physical impairments
Modification of task or assistance required	no	minimal to moderate	significant	Does the child require assistance or environmental modification to achieve an **age appropriate skill** of concern?
CLINICAL				

DECISION MAKING				
ANALYTICAL COMPLEXITY	low	moderate	high	Analysis of occupational profile, data from assessments and consideration of treatment options---**think in terms of wide ranging concerns and treatment options**

Every criteria or higher must be met within the selected CPT code

Courtesy of The Small Patient Practice, 2nd Ed., 2017

A one page download of this chart is available on www.smallpatientpractice.com

User: small

Password: practice

To XXX
Attn: EXAMPLE PATIENT GROUP
PO BOX 12345
CITY, State 88888-2345

Subject: INCORRECT PROCESSING OF CLAIM
Patient: Little Boy
DOB: 01/01/2002
Member ID: MED54321
Dates of Service: 6/3/2017-6/24/2017
Claim ID: Listed on the EOB (copy attached)

TO WHOM IT MAY CONCERN:
                          This is to notify you that you have incorrectly processed an
outpatient physical therapy claim for the above stated patient and dates of service.
You have arbitrarily changed the status of the claim from outpatient physical
therapy to home health care services.

        I billed the services listed according to CPT coding rules and CMS instructions.
Federal law requires that 'the parties shall comply with all applicable Medicare laws,
regulations and CMS instructions'.

        Medicare Benefit Policy manual, Pub 100-2, Chapter 15, 230.4 states
outpatient therapy services should be furnished in the therapist's or group's office
or in the patient's home.

        I am a private practice physical therapist and am in no way affiliated with a
home health care agency.

        Please review the attached claim and make the appropriate corrections in a
timely manner. If you prefer that I bill for these services in an alternative manner,
please let me know.

        Thank you,

Therapist name, credentials,   address listed, phone

The Small Patient Practice

This was submitted by the United States Department of Health and Human Services

To all healthcare providers:

It is unlawful to routinely waive copayments, deductibles, coinsurances, or other patient responsibility payments.

This includes services deemed as "professional courtesy" and "TWIP's
- Take what insurance pays".

Absent financial hardship, a "good faith effort" must be made to collect all deductibles and co-payments due and owed.

Failure to comply makes you in violation of the Federal False Claims Act, Federal Anti-Kickback Statute, and the Federal and State Insurance Fraud Laws.

Failure to comply may result in civil money penalties (CMP) in accordance with the new provision section 1128 A(a)(5) of the Health Insurance Portability and Accountability Act of 1996 [section 231(h) of HIPAA].

For any questions please contact:
Office of Inspector General
Department of Health and Human Services:
-by phone: 202 619-1343
-by fax: 202 260-8512
-by email: paffairs@oig.hhs.gov
-by mail: Office of Inspector General
Office of Public Affairs
Department of Health and Human Services
Room 5541 Cohen Building
333 Independence Avenue, S.W.
Washington, D.C. 20201
Joel Schaer
Office of Counsel to the Inspector General
202 619-0089

Appendix M

Bill to:
Patient or Parent Name
3345 Friendly Drive
City, State   zip code

Pay to:
Your company name (your name)
Your street address
City, State   zip code
Phone:

Statement of Payments and Balances

Today's Date:
Patient Name:
Insurance:

Type of service:
Service provider:

Date of Service	Allowable Charges	Insurance Paid	Patient Deductible	Co-pay/ Co-Ins	Balance owed	Total Owed

Message: You can give any explanation or message here

Appendix N

Policy: Parent Presence During Physical Therapy Sessions

Infants and toddlers with impairments requiring physical therapy, also require an alliance between the parents and therapist. Most therapy sessions include demonstrations of techniques to parents so that they can follow through with observed and recommended activities.   Your child requires your assistance in order to progress.

If you work full time and have a regular child care provider, you may provide permission for your child care provider to be present in your place for some of the physical therapy sessions.

THERAPIST will make every effort to schedule sessions for a time that is convenient to one or both parents and when your child is most ready to work.

THERAPIST is not affiliated with a Home Health Care Agency and so if your child receives Home Health Care nursing services, you should understand that THERAPIST does not have a contractual relationship which would allow her to extend her services through nurse care providers who are not related to your child. Nurse care providers are certainly welcome to be present and observe therapy sessions and they can follow through with any recommended activities that you request. Nurse care providers should not be a substitute for your presence.

THERAPIST is a working mom and understands the challenges related to meeting scheduled appointments. If you cannot be present for your child's physical therapy session please cancel your appointment within 24 hours of the scheduled time.

You may leave a message on her cell phone at 123-4567.

I have read and understand THERAPIST's policy regarding parental presence during physical therapy sessions.   _____Parent Signature

I give _____ permission to attend physical therapy sessions with my child when neither of his/her parents are available to attend. Jeanine Colburn has my permission to share any relevant medical information necessary to provide service and instruct my representative in home exercise programming

_____/_____Parent signature/ date

Child's Name: DOB:

Memorandum of Understanding

ADULT AGREEMENT TO ACCOMPANY MINOR

DURING MEDICAL PROCEDURE

I have agreed to accompany _____
when he/she receives Physical Therapy treatments with THERAPIST

I understand that I am expected to follow through with recommended activities and I will share any advice and recommendations with the child's parents.

I understand that if THERAPIST observes a health concern of major significance or importance, she will contact the parents directly for consultation.

_____   Date: _____
signature

GLOSSARY AND DEFINITIONS

Adaptive equipment—any equipment or device, including Assistive Technology, that helps a person achieve daily functional activities, including but not limited to moving, speaking and sitting.

Assistive technology—equipment considered to be technological in nature that helps a person achieve daily functional activities.

Automated programs—computer based programs which are programmed to recognize and match particular billing codes for payment.

Balance billing—billing the patient the difference between the amount allowed by the patient's Healthcare Insurance and the amount you billed. This is usually not allowed if you are a network provider.

Benefit plan—the healthcare benefits allowed by the patient's healthcare plan

Business license—a state license to own and run a business

Care coordination—the sharing of relevant information and coordinating care between providers of one patient

Centers for Medicare and Medicaid—A U.S.Department of Health and Human Services website, http://www.cms.gov/

Claim form—the form used to bill Healthcare Insurance, Medicaid and other payers. The name of the form used for outpatient, PT, OT and Speech services is Form CMS-1500

Clinic—a rehabilitation setting used to provide outpatient PT, OT and Speech Therapy services

Clinical judgment—the professional health care provider's determination of a patient's needs based upon evaluation, testing and professional opinion

CMS—The acronym used for Centers for Medicare and Medicaid Services http://www.cms.gov/

Cognitive disorder—a disorder which affects intellectual thinking and reasoning

Coinsurance—a patient portion of payment for services (usually a percentage) required by the patient's Health Insurance plan

Condition descriptor—a word or phrase which describes a patient's condition. For medical billing the descriptor is assigned an ICD-10 code.

Copayment—a patient portion of payment for services (usually a fixed amount) required by the patient's health insurance plan

Co-treatment—concurrent treatment of a patient by two or more therapists

CPT—Current Procedural Terminology

Current Procedural Terminology—codes which report medical provider procedures and services

Deductible—refers to the annual amount the patient must pay toward medical services before the health insurance plan pays for services

Diagnosis—a label attached to a patient's medical condition

Disability—a measurement of a person's function with relation to activities and environmental factors as determined by the ICF (International Classification of Functioning, Disability and Health)

DOB—date of birth

Duplication of services—similar services provided by different providers to the same patient

Dysphagia—difficulty in swallowing

Early Intervention Program—a partially federally funded program under Part C of IDEA (Individuals with Disabilities Education Act)

EI—Early Intervention

Electronic billing—Medical billing online

Electronic documentation and billing program—a program designed to allow the healthcare provider to document and maintain patient records and to bill electronically using one system

EOB-- Explanation of Benefits

Expected Outcome—the expected result of patient treatment

Explanation of Benefits—a document provided by the healthcare payer, describing services billed and paid

Form CMS-1500—the claim form used for the medical billing of outpatient physical therapy, occupational therapy and speech therapy services

Fraud—intentional deception or misrepresentation that the individual knows to be untrue, knowing that the deception results in benefit to himself or some other person

Health Care Reform—this term refers to the 2010 Affordable Health Care Act

Health Insurance Administrator—the office which manages the patient's health insurance plan

Health Insurance Portability and Accountability Act—protects health insurance coverage for workers and their families when they change or lose their jobs, establishes national standards for electronic healthcare transactions and national identifiers for providers, health insurance plans, and employers. Provides rules and guidelines for protection of patient health information.

Healthcare payer—the payer of healthcare services, including public and private health insurance, state and federal health plans

Healthcare plan—the patient's healthcare coverage, including benefits, exemptions, coinsurance, deductibles

Healthcare policy—the product used by the patient for healthcare coverage

Hemiparesis—weakness on one side of the body

High volume practice—a rehabilitation service with large numbers of patients and usually multiple providers

HIPAA-- Health Insurance Portability and Accountability Act

Home based outpatient therapy—outpatient rehabilitation provided in the patient's home/natural environment

Home Healthcare Agency—an agency which provides healthcare services to patients who are homebound, usually for medical reasons

Home office—an office in the provider's home

ICD 10 codes---International Classification of Disease, 10th Revision, Clinical Modification diagnosis codes

Impairment—a condition which impairs but does not obstruct function

Incorporate—a legal term for formation of a legal corporation

In-network—refers to a provider who has a contract with the healthcare payer

Insurance company—refers to a public or private healthcare insurance company

Insurance coverage year—each healthcare plan has a defined year of coverage. Patient deductibles and benefits fall within that defined year and start over again when the new coverage year begins.

Insurance plan—see Healthcare plan

IRS—Internal Revenue Service

Joint hypermobility—unusual looseness of the human body's joints

Liability Insurance—insurance for the professional healthcare provider which covers costs in the event of a professionally related incident

Long term patient—a patient requiring services which expand over a prolonged period of time (usually more than 6 months)

Medicaid—a state controlled healthcare plan typically for low income recipients and people with disabilities

Medical ID—an identification number assigned to a health benefits recipient

Medical payer—any payer of healthcare services

Medical record—a medical file which contains a patient's medical information

Medically necessary—a treatment which is necessary to resolve, improve or arrest the patient's medical condition

Medicare—a federal healthcare plan for the elderly

Medicare policy manual—a publicly accessible document which includes all policies around covered benefits for Medicare recipients, available at http://www.cms.gov/

National Provider Identifier—a unique identification number for covered health care providers intended for use in administrative and financial transactions

Natural environment—environment which is typical and natural to the patient

Neighborhood covenants—certain restrictions associated with the use of property or land within a community

Network contract—a contract between a provider and a healthcare payer

Network provider—a provider who is contracted to provide services with a particular Healthcare payer

Non-network provider—a provider who provides healthcare services without a network contract

NPI-- National Provider Identifier

Out-of-network—services received from a provider who does not have a contract with the payer

Outpatient therapy—rehabilitation services not associated with hospital care, skilled nursing facility or home health care

Paper bills—bills submitted on a paper form, usually by mail

Pathology—a clear disorder related to a medical condition

Patient privacy—the patient's right to prevent release of information regarding his medical condition to anyone who is not directly involved in his medical care

Pediatric rehabilitation—the treatment of children with medical conditions requiring physical rehabilitation or habilitation

Physician referral—a physician request for services

Primary care provider—the patient's primary physician

Prior authorization—permission from the healthcare payer to allow payment for services

Privacy notice—the provider's written policy describing what patient information will be shared and how

Private Practice—a privately owned practice

Privately funded plans—health insurance plans funded by the employee's company, but managed by a health insurance administrator

Professional association—an association dedicated to a particular profession

Professional designation—abbreviations or acronyms associated with a qualified provider of service

Professional organization—see 'professional association'

Prognosis—predictive outcome

Progressive disorders—disorders which are known to cause aspects of patient's condition to progressively decline

Referral—request for service

School based services—services provided in public schools as part of a student's IEP (Individualized Education Plan)

Self funded plans—see 'privately funded plans'

Self referral—the patient requests services directly from the provider

Solo practitioner—a provider who works alone

Standardized developmental evaluation—an evaluation tool which compares a child's developmental skills to those of same aged peers and which results in a score with standardized reliability

Timed code—a CPT code which has time associated with its use

TRICARE—the healthcare program serving military service members, retirees and their families

Untimed code—a CPT code which has no associated time guidelines or restrictions

Visit—healthcare provider contact with a patient which includes treatment

WNL—within normal limits

Index

Adaptive equipment, 97

AOTA, 5, 25, 59,77

APTA, 22,25,59

ASHA, 25,59

Authorization, 14, 16, 19, 22, 45, 52, 84, 99

Benefits, 10,23

Business expenses, 112

Centers for Medicare and Medicaid/

CMS, 4, 6, 21, 25, 34, 36, 37, 42, 43, 44, 45, 46, 52, 55, 60, 87

Coinsurance, 10, 15, 83

Copayment, 10, 15, 88, 89

Corrected claim, 47, 101

CPT code, 3, 9, 35, 49, 59, 60, 61, 68, 69, 76, 77, 79

Deductible, 13, 15, 88

Denials, 69, 99

Developmental delay, 27, 59, 92

Diagnosis, 29, 46, 49, 50, 56, 58, 92

Discharge note, 37

Down Syndrome, 9, 47, 57

Durable medical equipment, 30, 97

Dysphagia, 29, 58, 99

Early Intervention, 4, 9, 24, 26, 55, 92, 111

EOB/Explantion of Benefits, 10, 23, 81, 82, 85

Health Care Reform, 4

HIPAA, 3, 4, 8, 18, 22, 45, 60, 68, 105-108

Home exercise, 64, 65, 94, 95

Home healthcare agency, 84

ICD 10 code, 3, 9, 55-59

Incorporation, 7

Liability, 6, 7, 111

Liability insurance, 6, 8, 112

Licensure requirements, 6, 37, 111, 113

Medicaid, 4, 6, 12, 15, 25, 44, 46, 67, 68, 87, 103

Medical necessity, 25, 26, 34, 53, 92, 99, 100

Modifier code, 65, 68

Network, 8, 9, 10,13-16, 20, 23, 51, 53, 82, 83, 88, 100, 101

NPI, 6, 7, 8, 51, 52

Office Ally, 41

Outpatient therapy, 9, 12, 34, 41, 42, 84 101

Permission to bill, 20, 21, 45, 47

Physician referral, 14, 19, 20, 25, 38

Physician referral, 20, 21, 27, 41, 88

Place of Service, 48

Plan of Care, 25, 94, 95

Privacy Notice, 21, 22

Privately funded plans, 11

Progress report, 20, 33, 34, 36

Progressive disorder, 75, 94, 95

Rule of 8, 60-63

School based services, 101

Sensory integration, 27, 93

Service provider change, 38

Signature on file, 21, 46

Standardized developmental assessment, 28

Timed codes, 35, 49, 60-63, 66

Treatment note, 20, 34-37

Untimed codes, 35, 37, 50, 63, 66

Made in the USA
Middletown, DE
10 January 2021